Protecting Patients' Rights?

A comparative study of the ombudsman in healthcare

Edited by

Stephen Mackenney
Associate Director
Patient Experience
NHS Clinical Governance Support Team

and

Lars Fallberg
Chief Executive
Picker Scandinavia
Research Fellow
Nordic School of Public Health

Radcliffe Medical Press

Radcliffe Medical Press Ltd
18 Marcham Road
Abingdon
Oxon OX14 1AA
United Kingdom

www.radcliffe-oxford.com
The Radcliffe Medical Press electronic catalogue and online ordering facility.
Direct sales to anywhere in the world.

British Library Cataloguing in Publication Data

A catalogue record for this book is available from the British Library.

ISBN 1 85775 870 6

Typeset by Advance Typesetting Ltd, Oxfordshire
Printed and bound by TJ International Ltd, Padstow, Cornwall

Contents

List of contributors

Ioanna Arsenopoulou MD, MSc
General Director, Regional Health System of Dodecanese
Formerly, Senior Investigator, Office of the Greek Ombudsman

Gerald Bachinger
Spokesman, Austrian Arbeitsgemeinschaft Patientenanwalt (ARGE PA)

Lars Fallberg LLM
Chief Executive, Picker Scandinavia
Research Fellow, Nordic School of Public Health, Gothenberg

Eftichis Fitrakis LLB, LLM, PhD
Senior Investigator, Office of the Greek Ombudsman

Philip Giddings
Senior Lecturer in Politics, University of Reading
Co-Director, Centre for Ombudsman and Governance Studies, London

Galya M Hildesheimer LLM
Gertner Institute for Epidemiology & Health Policy Research, Tel Hashomer

Mervi Kattelus
Senior Adviser, Ministry of Social Affairs and Health, Helsinki

Stephen Mackenney MA(Cantab), BL
Associate Director, Patient Experience, NHS Clinical Governance Support Team

Olav Molven
Associate Professor, Diakonhjemmet College, Oslo

John Øvretveit
Professor of Health Policy and Management
Nordic School of Public Health, Gothenberg

Judit Sándor
Associate Professor of Law and Political Science
Central European University, Budapest

Carmel Shalev JSD
Gertner Institute for Epidemiology & Health Policy Research, Tel Hashomer

Introduction

*Lars Fallberg, Stephen Mackenney
and John Øvretveit*

'Ombudsman', originally a Swedish word, has come to mean many things to many people. It has been adopted in a number of countries over the years, as a term for an administrative system which acts to protect the interests of individual citizens who complain against an administrative system. How that protection manifests itself varies markedly from country to country, depending on many factors, not least the historical and cultural differences of each. This book aims to give an overview of the role of the Ombudsman – past, present and future – as it is in seven national systems where there are such differences in culture and history: Austria, Finland, Greece, Hungary, Israel, Norway and the UK.

Experts from each country have kindly contributed to this work, with a chapter from each describing their own national system. The approaches taken by each country that they describe likewise differ – from national to local and from adjudicator to individual representative. There are merits to all the systems along the scale, as inevitably one size does not fit all. This book examines in practical terms how each of the systems operates, and where from a national perspective reform would be desirable.

In this introduction, we seek to identify what objectively constitute the key characteristics of an Ombudsman. We also open the debate on where an Ombudsman system of any complexion could play a greater role by expanding beyond the boundaries of individual complaint resolution and influencing quality improvement more generally.

After the contributions of the seven national authors, we seek by way of conclusion to analyse the key advantages of each system, and thereby to extract the best components. Building on our initial suggestion for a wider role in quality improvement, we offer at the close of the book some overall proposals which might inform thinking around future reforms and the introduction of similar systems elsewhere. Let us begin first of all with a brief description of the origins of the Ombudsman, and some of the most important aspects of its role.

The right to complain ...

It is human nature, in most circumstances, to want to react in some way and maybe even to complain when one feels that one has been subjected to an injustice, or to unfair treatment. The process of complaining has an additional purpose when an individual wants to send a message to decision-makers within an institution that an aspect of the way they work is unreasonable – for example in the field of healthcare services, waiting times or access to care.

In many social arenas – when among equals, in the course of a commercial transaction, or with many public sector services – people will generally feel both ready and able to complain. This is not always the case in the healthcare setting, where individuals will often rely on healthcare professionals in the most personal way for their own welfare and security. Traditional barriers created by the culture of institutionalised national healthcare and the awe inspired by the medical professional do still exist. While in some countries they are being gradually broken down as action to empower patients gathers momentum, we cannot yet escape the truism of 'doctor knows best'. Nor can we escape the fact that, administratively, it is often the case that the well-being of society may be given priority over what is best for an individual.

In the sphere of the rights of patients in healthcare systems, the right to complain and the right to appeal against a first instance decision on a complaint are viewed as part of the basic fabric of rights and obligations. By the same token, the existence of an effective complaints procedure is absolutely necessary to ensure that patients complaining against the violation of their rights can find redress.

Perhaps in the past the basic right to complain has not always been self-evident to patients, for the reasons given above. But increasingly in the course of recent decades in most western societies, systems have been introduced which make explicit the procedure for complaining, and which offer a formalised route for appeal and redress alongside traditional litigious channels.

... and a procedure for doing so

In most cases, complaints systems begin with processes internal to the healthcare institutions themselves. This approach in many ways is well justified: local problem resolution is often proven to be most effective, swift and desirable for both the complainant and the healthcare institution (as is well demonstrated, for example, in England). While the two parties are engaged face to face, there is an opportunity, outwith the scope of more antagonistic litigation, to:

* undertake a primary investigation
* confront underlying systemic or managerial problems within institutions directly
* offer an apology to the complainant for a wrong suffered (often no more than that is sought, though failure to provide it inevitably leads to an escalation of the complaint)
* mediate a solution.

However, these potential advantages can be the very cause of failure for a first instance complaints procedure: investigations may not be undertaken, or may be less than transparent to the complainant. Institutions may decide to take steps internally to rectify systemic problems, but are often highly defensive when asked to recognise publicly that such problems exist.

Most importantly, the whole procedure tends to require the persistence, energy and expertise of an individual or team in good health with all the necessary information resources at their fingertips. Complaints procedures have rarely been designed in a way that makes them simple, accessible, and expeditious from the complainant's perspective. It can take years for a complaint to be resolved to everyone's satisfaction, and sometimes this may never be the case. Of course, there are vexatious complainants in the field of healthcare as elsewhere, but these are never in the majority, and do not account for all unresolved cases. Genuine complainants need therefore also to be physically and mentally resilient enough to steer their case along the seemingly serpentine path set down by the institution they face. If necessary, they need also to be prepared to pursue one or more appeals to find the right solution for them.

Support for complainants

As a result of the tortuousness of many complaints procedures, systems of advocacy and support for complainants, formal or informal, have begun to emerge. These seek in most cases to offer the basic knowledge and expertise for those who wish to complain: how best to initiate a complaint, the choice of which route to follow, and what to expect from the procedure as the administrative wheels begin to turn. At the other end of the spectrum, the need has also been recognised for effective appeals procedures. These should be, and be seen to be, independent, rigorous in their investigation, from an unbiased perspective and unafraid to draw unpopular conclusions.

These needs are most certainly real to patients: to be supported through the various steps of a difficult procedure; to have an articulate and detached mouthpiece when dealing with highly personal and emotive issues; and to see an independent figure leading the way in adjudication. And the full range of this spectrum – from the local on-site advocate to the national impartial appeals investigator – has been in one form or another introduced under the aegis of a patient or healthcare Ombudsman.

The origin of the Ombudsman function

The word 'Ombudsman' has its origin in Sweden and is used to identify someone who has the rights and powers to speak on behalf of someone else, for example in court or in other situations. 'Ombudsman' was introduced by the Swedish King Karl XII about 300 years ago. After King Karl XII had lost a battle against the Russians in Poltava in 1709 he went to Turkey and stayed there for several years before returning to Sweden. The absence of the King created turbulence in the Swedish state administration and a government office was created to take care of the administration of the country. The highest-ranking officer at the government office was called Ombudsman and he was labelled Ombudsman of the King during the King's absence from the country.

Since the days of King Karl XII a number of national Ombudsmen institutions have been developed in Sweden. Among the earlier ones were the Chancellor of Justice (1713), Parliamentary Ombudsman (1809), the Consumer Ombudsman (1971), the Children's Ombudsman (1993), the Ombudsman against Ethnic Discrimination (1986), the Equal Opportunities Ombudsman (1980) and the Disability Ombudsman (1994). The latest addition to the exclusive 'club' of Ombudsmen is the Ombudsman against Discrimination as a result of Sexual Orientation (1999).

In Sweden there are several similarities as well as differences between these thematic Ombudsmen depending on the interest they are designed to protect. The body to which all the different Ombudsmen institutions are accountable is, with one exception, the Swedish government. The exception is the Parliamentary Ombudsman, who is accountable to Parliament. Any citizen can turn to the Parliamentary Ombudsman if he or she has been treated wrongly or unjustly by a public authority or an official employed by the civil service or local government.

The legal basis for the actions of the Ombudsmen also differs: again it is the Parliamentary Ombudsmen whose role, function and powers are regulated by the constitution whilst the powers of other Ombudsmen are defined in legislation. The functions and powers of the Chancellor of Justice are, however, mixed. The legal basis for the Chancellor of Justice is drawn partly from the constitution, partly from legislation, which place this particular Ombudsman in a special category from the others. The actions of the 'thematic' Ombudsmen are to some extent based upon human rights. The Equal Opportunities Ombudsman, the Ombudsman against Ethnic Discrimination and the Ombudsman against Discrimination as a result of Sexual Orientation primarily base their activities on the principle of non-discrimination.

The work of the Parliamentary Ombudsman and the Chancellor of Justice are strictly focused on the supervision of governmental authorities and their respect for, and actions in accordance with, the law. The other Ombudsmen are more engaged in whether specific requirements in legislation or international commitments have been fulfilled. Counselling, influencing public opinion and providing information to citizens in general may fulfil these tasks. A conclusive difference between the Parliamentary Ombudsman and the Chancellor of Justice on the one side and the thematic Ombudsmen on the other is that the latter are primarily engaged in policy issues and are focused on the promotion of their respective goals.

The legal powers of the different Ombudsmen vary. The Parliamentary Ombudsman and the Chancellor of Justice both have the right to decide on issuing a fine if a defined task is not fulfilled and also to decide on public prosecution. The Consumer Ombudsman, the Ombudsman against Ethnic Discrimination, the Equal Opportunities Ombudsman, the Disability Ombudsman and the Ombudsman against Discrimination as a result of Sexual Orientation may decide on issuing a fine. They may also plead their cause in a civil court. In addition the Disability Ombudsman is also empowered to invite parties to negotiations under which such parties are required to be present under the law. All Ombudsmen are required to make a report of their activities each year. The Parliamentary Ombudsman has to report to Parliament while the others give their reports to the government.

It is from these roots that the various administrative systems around the globe entitled 'Ombudsman' have spread. Though Sweden itself has not developed the thematic role of its Ombudsmen specifically into healthcare, the principles and models show themselves to be readily transferable. We shall now look at how other countries have adapted these principles in the sphere of healthcare services.

The seedlings of the Patient Ombudsman in Finland, the UK and the USA

Since the 'birth' of the Ombudsman Institute in Sweden at the beginning of the 18th century a number of countries have imported the Ombudsman Institution.

Several countries have developed the function with different powers, depending on local traditions, values and the history of the country in question. The development of a Patient Ombudsman, however, emerged to start with over the course of the last two decades of the last century. The United States is one example, although the term Ombudsman has not been as frequently used as the term Patient Advocate. In the early 1970s one of the leading researchers in the USA in terms of patients' rights, George Annas, proposed a patient rights' advocate. Some years later, several American states developed some version of a patient bill of rights including a patient rights' advocate. According to Annas a patient rights advocate is 'a person whose job is to help patients exercise the rights outlined in the state's or institution's Patient Bill of Rights'. He stresses that one of the most critical characteristics of the advocate is that he represents the patient, the reason being that the goal is to enhance the patient's position in making decisions, not to encourage the patient to follow facility routine or to 'behave'.

In the UK, the Ombudsman referred to as the Health Service Commissioner emerged out of the function of the Parliamentary Commissioner in 1973. The function was established for England, for Scotland and for Wales, along the lines of the Parliamentary Commissioner for Administration scheme but with clinical judgement excluded.

In Finland, the law on the status and rights of a patient, enacted in 1992, introduced for the first time a Patient Ombudsman. However, instead of having a national institution, hundreds of Patient Ombudsmen were appointed across Finland, often nurses or social workers working as Ombudsmen in addition to their normal functions. Since then, several Patient Ombudsman schemes have emerged across Europe.

Features central to an effective Patient Ombudsman system

Owing to the existence of significant variations in the role and functions of Patient Ombudsmen in existing systems, it is difficult to define what the necessary features of an effective system are. However, to some degree the functions of a Patient Ombudsman are the same as with an effective complaints system. This has much to do with the relationship of trust, which must exist between a patient and the party responsible for receiving and dealing with the complaint.

Impartiality and independence

A necessary characteristic of an effective Patient Ombudsman institution is the complete impartiality of the office and its employees. Impartiality is best demonstrated and reinforced by administrative or statutory independence, though this is not always essential, depending on the role of the Ombudsman and whether other means of underpinning impartiality exist. Such independence might be organisational as well as financial in terms of staff salaries and future office budgets. We examine these distinctions somewhat more below.

Impartiality should also represent a demonstrable facet of any subsequent investigation into a complaint as well as the recommendations coming as the result of such an investigation. These recommendations should not be influenced by paternalistic approaches or traditional views, but should focus on the rights of the individual in combination with the quality improvement of the institutions involved.

Impartiality and independence: the stakeholder's perspective

A complaint will always involve a number of conflicting interests. There is not just the patient as user of healthcare services, and the healthcare institution as service provider. In publicly provided health services, the perspective of the funding organisation will also be involved (whether in the form of the national or regional health department, or county or municipal service commissioning body). Individual healthcare professionals, who will often be the real focus of the complaint, will also have a keen personal interest from the point of view of their professional reputation and integrity. Other onlookers, such as quality audit departments and patient representative organisations, will also have something to say. Many stakeholders will regard their argument as compelling and their perspective as of greater importance than all others.

With so many conflicting stakeholder interests, the question then arises as to how far any individual fulfilling the function of Patient Ombudsman can or should be wholly independent of the system in which they operate. If seen to be sympathising too closely with any one perspective, the Patient Ombudsman risks drawing criticism from competing quarters which it may be difficult to deflect. In essence the answer seems to be a matter of degree: certainly one who seeks to act as adjudicator of a complaint will need to be, and be seen to be, independent and impartial. Impartiality should also be a prerequisite for anyone holding themselves up to be a true adviser and advocate of the complainant: excessive personal involvement will inevitably mar the quality of advice and support. But should such an individual be independent – whether statutorily, by employment or both? To find a true answer to the question of independence requires an analysis of the real role played by the Patient Ombudsman, and the cultural backdrop of the healthcare system in which they work: the subject for the rest of this book.

Competence

It is not enough to appoint anyone interested in patients' rights issues to a post in a Patient Ombudsman's office. It is always possible to find people dedicated to doing the right thing but they will often lack proper training in how to resolve conflicts and deal with different stakeholders and their respective interests. To gain the respect of patients as well as healthcare professionals it is important for officers working in the Patient Ombudsman's office to have sufficient training in all issues which might represent causes for someone to complain. Often, but not always, it is also useful to have someone with clinical experience, who understands the language of healthcare professionals. Legal training is also needed, as a Patient Ombudsman may have to deal with conflicts that could be taken to court or require some kind of semi-legal settlement between the parties.

Powers

The Ombudsman needs powers in order to be able to command the respect of the various different stakeholders. Since respect should not necessarily have to result from the threat of legal remedies and sanctions – and would not, in the case of the Ombudsman – we need to analyse what other kinds of administrative powers are respected by others. In some countries an Ombudsman's office will command respect simply if their investigations result in just and fair opinions. In others, this needs to be backed by a power to sanction wrongdoers, which makes an Ombudsman's office similar to any supervising authority. In any case, it is important to use the principle of proportionality in that an Ombudsman's office should not acquire greater force or powers than is needed in each national situation. Too few powers could create an institution without proper credibility and whose judgements are repeatedly disregarded by others. Too many powers could present a perverse incentive for healthcare staff – preventing them from doing the right thing for fear of punishment if they do something wrong.

A systematic approach

Complaints are a useful tool to create changes in any system producing services. However, a good evidence base is essential to be able to convince someone that they need to change their professional behaviour after a long career in health-care. To gather such evidence, it is crucial that all complaints are handled in a systematic way, that they are identified, documented, categorised and analysed. When an analysis has been carried out, the resulting conclusions need to be presented to the relevant healthcare professional or manager responsible for quality improvement at the unit in question. Proposals for change will have a much greater chance of successful implementation if they are presented as scientific evidence based upon systematic information gathering followed by a proper analysis.

The Ombudsman and quality improvement

The rest of this introduction considers one of the objectives of most Ombudsman schemes and one which is likely to play a greater role in the future. It addresses the question, 'how can Ombudsmen best contribute to improving the quality of health services overall?' This is an important question for Ombudsmen, as their development will depend on making a greater contribution to improving quality, not just on how well they handle individual complaints. It is also an important question for healthcare organisations, as they often fail to recognise and use the help which Ombudsmen can offer in driving quality improvement.

First we consider features of the modern approach to quality improvement. Then we consider whether and how Ombudsmen can be part of the systematic approach to quality improvement, which many organisations and countries are establishing. The chapter ends with recommendations and questions for both Ombudsmen and for health services to make more use of Ombudsmen to improve quality.

Modern quality improvement

The authors and others believe that Ombudsman schemes can have a greater role in reducing the incidence of adverse events, suffering and costs for future patients. Often health services and Ombudsmen have not recognised the valuable part which such schemes can play in this respect. However, the modern approach to quality improvement makes it easier for Ombudsmen to play a greater part. Two changes in how we think about quality are particularly important: a change in the way we understand the cause of errors and a change in attitudes towards quality problems.

From 'complaints' and 'mistakes' to 'concerns' and 'adverse events'

The first is a change in thinking about the cause of 'complaints' and 'mistakes'. The traditional view is that the source of quality is the individual professional practitioner. A patient complaint is likely to be made either because the professional's 'bedside manner' or social skills were poor, which is not serious, or because there was a medical error or mistake due to an individual's incompetence or laziness. The defensiveness with which complaints are viewed is not surprising, given the traditional education and socialisation of health professionals and also the need which both patients and professionals have to believe in the professional's omnipotence.

The modern approach to quality does not use the terms 'error', 'mistake', or 'complaint', but instead, 'adverse event', 'mishap', or 'concern'. This is not to downgrade the seriousness of the event. Rather it is to avoid automatically viewing the event as being caused by an individual professional's oversight or negligence.

Quality problems are viewed as being caused by the poor organisation of a 'system of care'. Most systems of care are organised in such a way as to unintentionally cause an adverse event to occur sooner or later. One US hospital discovered that there were 94 steps from ordering a medication for an inpatient to the patient taking the medication. These 94 steps had to be successfully completed for each of the 12–15 different medications which each patient was taking. In a system like this errors will occur even when all professionals are working at their best. In some cases, errors are more likely if professionals are conscientious and follow the system carefully. The outcome could not be otherwise, given how the system was organised.

The modern approach to quality is to change the way the healthcare system is organised so as to reduce the chance of adverse events occurring in the future and to improve the patient's experience and clinical outcomes. There are many different quality methods, which are now being used by ordinary doctors, nurses and administrative employees to analyse and change the system.

Change in attitude and culture

For working practices to change and for quality to improve there has to be a change in attitudes. This is the second change which is taking place, largely for two reasons. First, as a result of increasing awareness of the problems inherent in systems of care, professionals are recognising that complaints and errors are often not their fault as individuals and are becoming less defensive. Organisations and laws are making it easier for employees to report their concerns. Second, more employees are learning and using methods to analyse systems of care and make changes to these systems: they are learning that they can take control over these error-producing systems and do something to prevent problems in the future.

Although they are being promoted by professionals and government, it would be wrong to imply that these two changes in thinking and attitude are widespread: they are just beginning. Many patients – and Ombudsmen – still view quality problems as only the result of insensitive or incompetent individuals rather than being partially or wholly caused by poor organisation of systems of care. For professionals it takes time to learn and apply the methods. Changing healthcare organisation to make it safer and produce a better experience for patients takes time, especially changing the way two or more services relate. Although many managers recognise the importance of quality, they often know little about the methods to achieve it. Nor do they necessarily have the skills to manage change to support the clinical professionals in their improvement work. The Ombudsman may be welcomed here, but getting effective change into systems is more difficult.

How the Ombudsman can help health services to improve quality

The way Ombudsmen have influenced quality in the past is largely through health services fearing becoming a subject of their attention. However, the threat of being found not to have followed laws or professional standards is of limited effectiveness for improving quality. The Ombudsman upholds rights and provides a necessary safeguard, but also needs to adopt the modern approach to quality: indeed to be part of the movement advocating a more widespread use of these approaches. Their motto should be 'We do not seek revenge, only to revise the system which caused this problem'.

How can they do this? Three ways are: to apply quality methods to their own service; to encourage health services to develop their own feedback systems; and to aggregate and analyse individual complaints data.

A better quality Ombudsman service

The Ombudsman provides a service to patients. As in many other services, Ombudsmen wish to provide a better service: to be quicker in dealing with complaints and to give more attention and time to each individual. Delays in handling complaints often make it more difficult not only to investigate the complaint but to make use of the investigation to improve the service in future: individuals or organisations may have changed radically since the time of the complaint. How, then, can Ombudsmen improve their service without extra personnel?

There is a case for more resources, but there is also room for improvements in efficiency, which allow a better service to patients. Ombudsmen can use process analysis and other quality methods to reduce unnecessary delays and costs. Using these methods to improve their own service also allows Ombudsmen to learn about these methods. This knowledge will be necessary in the future to work with health service personnel to improve healthcare.

Ombudsmen also need to consider the service which they provide to health services as a type of 'customer service': can they improve the quality of the feedback which they give, and the way in which they give the feedback? Quality methods include methods for finding out what health services most value and want from the Ombudsman.

Promoting health service patient feedback systems

Many health services do not seek feedback from either patients or professionals about quality issues, or use it to prevent problems. Many do not have easy-to-use first-stage internal complaints collection and resolution systems or ways for employees to report quality concerns or hazards. Many make complaining difficult, lose valuable learning opportunities and cause those patients who want to pursue the matter to go elsewhere. This usually costs the service more than an effective internal system.

Ombudsmen are the experts in complaints. They have experience about what causes complaints and knowledge about ways to collect and resolve complaints. They can give health services advice about how to develop their systems. Ombudsmen could also review or audit a service's complaints system, either offering this as a service or having this as an additional duty. At present resources and other constraints prevent Ombudsmen from extending their role in this way, but they can advocate for better internal complaints systems – if only to reduce unnecessary work for themselves.

Aggregating individual data

The Ombudsman's focus is on the individual and on the past. Past 'adverse events' provide important data for the detective work of locating the underlying cause of errors in the system. Often the system causes are easier to detect if data about many individual errors is aggregated: this makes it possible to see recurring patterns which are not visible at the level of the individual case. By not aggregating these individual data we are missing the opportunity to detect the underlying causes. It is not, however, a duty of Ombudsmen to carry out systematic analyses of this type, although they do make reports which usually involve a less systematic reflection on common problems.

Another obstacle to system problem identification is that patients can report their concerns and complaints to many different bodies. This in itself is not a problem: there is a case for having a variety of channels for complaints and different mechanisms for dealing with them. The problem for systems improvement is that all of the patient complaints are not brought together in a way which allows the problem patterns to be recognised.

There are two ways forward here. First, Ombudsmen could develop systems which allow them to enter details about individual cases and to analyse these data to find patterns which show recurring problems. To some extent many Ombudsmen do this, but not always in a systematic way and as one of their core responsibilities.

Second, a way needs to be found of collecting from all complaints handling systems certain data about each complaint, which can then be used to detect system problems. There is a need to document all the complaints made to different agencies about each health service. Each agency will need to provide certain data about each case so that an analysis can be carried out of all complaints to reveal patterns which would otherwise go unrecognised.

This raises a number of questions. Should the Ombudsman role expand to perform these analyses, not just for its own cases but for all complaints? Is this work better done by another organisation? If others do it, will Ombudsmen be less likely to enter the required up-to-date information for each case? As with individual cases, the quicker the analysis then the more useful the data are to the service.

Conclusions

Much can be learned from the different Ombudsmen schemes which have developed. It is clear that the Ombudsman has an important role in healthcare systems. One view is that their primary purpose is to support, serve and protect the individual patient, and this has certainly been their focus in the past. Currently, resources and remit require Ombudsmen to concentrate on individual complaints about past treatment. But it is also clear that their future role will include a greater emphasis on improving health-service quality. This chapter proposed that the data about and experience with individuals are wasted if they are not used to enable health services to change the way they provide patient care for the better. In the past Ombudsmen have been ahead of the capacity of health services to use their input. However, more and more health services are using modern quality methods and changing attitudes so that there is now an opportunity for Ombudsmen to make a greater contribution in this area. To do so Ombudsmen themselves need to learn and use quality methods to improve their own services to both patients and health-care services.

This discussion leads to a set of recommendations for increasing the contribution of Ombudsmen to improving healthcare quality, which are considered at the conclusion of this book. But first, it is helpful to develop an understanding of the practical systems that already exist, and how far they work within these parameters.

CHAPTER 1

The Patient Ombudsman System in Austria

Gerald Bachinger

'We don't look for culprits, we look for satisfying solutions for patients'*

Introduction and overview

The Ombudsman system in Austria

In Austria the Ombudsman system has been in place for a number of decades. The first steps were taken in the field of general administration in order to support citizens and protect them from intervention by the state. This institution ('Volksanwalt' – the People's Attorney, or PA) has had and still has extensive general competence. In the field of public health 'patients' representatives' were founded, with special powers, equipment and staff. This structural development took place along with an expansion and deepening of patient rights along with increased awareness in government, in parliamentary representation and among the population generally. This arose in the context of increased importance being accorded to patients' rights within Austria's legal system.

Supportive organisations for patients

It soon became clear, however, that the creation and expansion of patients' rights alone was not sufficient. It proved necessary to provide more information for patients to avail themselves of their rights. In addition to the existence of rights, a supportive organisation was also necessary.

In a constitutional state like Austria lawyers and courts offer legal representation that can by no means cover in their entirety the complex and diverse themes to be found in many complaints cases within the public health system. This solely legally-focused support is only concerned with traditional malpractice and cannot offer

---

* This is the most important 'motto' of the PAs; it epitomises the purpose of the work of the PAs. It should be made clear that PAs act neither as judge, nor jury, nor executioner.

communication, mediation etc. However, these latter aspects are often more important to patients than legal support. Court procedures are protracted, often over several years and often involve a good deal of personal commitment and high financial risk for the patient. These last two aspects in particular have led to patients not instigating legal action for their causes. Meantime, making access to legal rights clearer, and providing other aid, has not necessarily helped to alleviate the problem.

The benefit of the system of *Patientenanwälte* (PAs)

This practical experience eventually led to the establishment of an extensive complaint management system – the independent Ombudsman system – within the Austrian health system. In some states this institution is called 'representation of patients' (*Patientenvertretungen*), in other states, 'PAs'. This independent Ombudsman system, which is not subject to any external direction, has been well tested. Three points illustrate the levels of recognition and appreciation of this system:

1 the population's increasing use of patients' representatives (PAs)
2 the consultation of PAs as experts and advisers in decision making by political authorities in the field of health. This is because PAs are able to draw upon their experience of close contact with patients and their relatives and healthcare professionals
3 there are currently no private organisations offering a similar service.

History

Carinthia and Upper Austria were the first to found a PA and patient representative system respectively, in 1991, followed in 1992 by the Vienna PA and the Styrian patient representative, in 1994 by the Lower Austrian PA, in 1995 by the Salzburg patient representative and in 1996 by the patient representative for the district hospitals of the Tyrol. The last additions were Vorarlberg's PA in 1999 and Burgenland's in 2001. In 1993 a federal law was enacted requiring all the *Länder* (the federal states of Austria) to employ PAs. This requirement by the federal legislature was recognised in different ways by different states. PAs and patient representatives therefore have a common base but different structures.

Different regional structures

Differences can be seen in denomination; in responsibilities – either covering the overall health and social care system, or just certain areas of health, specifically hospitals (*see* Table 1.1); and in structures and organisation – all PAs and representatives are established for the entire state except for the Tyrol, where patient representatives are established separately in each hospital or for several hospitals together.

Table 1.1   Variations in competencies and responsibility

State	Hospitals	Nursing home	Licensed medical practitioner	Social insurance	Life saving services	Organisation
Burgenland	X	X	X	X	X	central
Carinthia	X		X			central
Lower Austria	X	X	X	X	X	central
Salzburg	X					central
Styria	X	X				central
Tyrol	X					decentral
Upper Austria	X					central
Vienna	X	X	X	X	X	central
Vorarlberg	X	X	X	X	X	central

All PAs are founded in law, at one level based on federal law (hospital laws), and then on one state law per federal state. Freedom from supervision and the independence of PAs are ensured by constitutional laws in each of the states. Having this independence, PAs can provide their patients with a guaranteed level of professional service in handling and supporting their cases.

Organisational structure

All PAs are established regionally, i.e. for the entire state (except for the Tyrol). However, in some states, hospitals have founded Ombudsmen voluntarily and without legal obligation, though this is rare. In the state of Tyrol, legally established PAs are locally competent for one or several hospitals.

Co-ordination throughout Austria

In the year 2000 a team (*Arbeitsgemeinschaft* = ARGE) of all PAs was established in order to overcome these differences and to enable more co-ordinated working.
   This ARGE pursues the following goals:

• promotion and development of patients' rights
• co-ordinated action within and between PAs
• exchange of information and experience
• further development and unification (where possible) of structures within PAs.

All PAs are members of this ARGE. The spokesman of the ARGE, at this time Dr Gerald Bachinger, is an elected officer.

Financing of the PAs

All PAs are publicly financed. They are employed by the state (except in Tyrol, where they are employees of the public hospitals), meaning that the state also takes on full responsibility for the work of the PA. The PAs are allocated an annual budget which consists of the staffing and non-staffing (materials etc) expenditure for the year. The staffing element of this will of course vary significantly according to the PAs' staff complement (the bigger the state, the higher the staffing levels). Non-staffing expenditure also varies, covering a wide range of items, such as costs for journeys, expert literature, advanced training, medical opinions sought, and for project work (e.g. projects on information for patients). Again the size of the state will determine expenditure – ranging in 2001 from €30 000 in Salzburg (½ m inhabitants, 7 hospitals), to around €140 000 in Lower Austria (½ m inhabitants, 27 public hospitals).

Overall responsibilities

Securing the rights of patients

The main responsibility of PAs is safeguarding and securing the rights and interests of patients. All PAs have competence for hospitals as a minimum and therefore handle complaints and defend patients' interests. Some PAs have produced brochures to advise patients about their rights and on the services offered. The PAs also run internet web pages which contain a good deal of information about patients' rights and the service of the PAs.

In terms of the competence of PAs, what is important is not where a patient's permanent home address is, but rather what the reason for, or origin of, the complaint is. For instance, the PA in Lower Austria is competent to deal with a complaint concerning a Lower Austrian hospital, even if the patient's permanent address is in a different federal state or abroad.

Extrajudicial settlement

PAs are service- and patient-orientated institutions that co-operate with staff in intra- and extra-mural healthcare areas. PAs look for extrajudicial solutions wherever possible rather than for legal judgements in favour of the patient. This duty is underpinned in state laws, which provide that the PAs should seek extrajudicial settlements. However, there are no codes of practice or single set of objectives for the work of the PAs which extrapolate from this, though civil jurisprudence is used to negotiate financial solutions e.g. in cases of malpractice.

The focal point and the most demanding activities for PAs lie in the examination, preparation and pursuit of cases to find extrajudicial solutions in cases of medical malpractice. Here PAs usually co-operate with doctors' liability insurers and hospitals and with the arbitration boards of the general medical councils. Suggested solutions have to be well supported in terms of argument and evidence owing to the principle that these extrajudicial proceedings are voluntary. Settlements are only possible when all parties concerned agree.

Patient compensation funds

For some years the introduction of a new compensation model was discussed in the context of improving the rights of the patient, with a view to introducing liability without fault. Different models were developed and discussed, but no specific model achieved full support, for the simple reason that the financing of any such new models was not possible and this remains the case.

In 2001 the functions and responsibilities of PAs were extended by the involvement of PAs in new forms of patient compensation. The funds are established in every federal state in Austria separately. In most of the states the funds are already regularised within state law and all of them have fixed rules of procedure. Generally this new initiative will lead to further improvements in the relationships between patients and hospitals, as there will now be the opportunity to seek compensation in cases of hardship. If the legal liability of a hospital is not clearly established, and if not offering compensation would be considered inequitable, damages can be covered in part by national compensation funds. The upper limit is €22 000, though this can be exceeded in special cases of hardship.

A commission of experts will examine the case and, if applicable, take steps for part of the patients' damages claim to be covered. Members of the commission vary from state to state, but generally include a jurist (e.g. a judge or a lawyer), a physician, a representative of patient self-help groups and the PA. In Lower Austria, Upper Austria and Salzburg the PA chairs the commission. Before referral to the commission, PAs have to examine whether, under compensation laws, full compensation would be possible, because these criteria would still have to be met for the purposes of a commission ruling.

Generally, the compensation fund is applicable in two types of case:

- there is a lack of evidence and so liability is not established for certain
- not all requirements for liability are met, but it would not be equitable to mitigate damages, because of the scale or rarity of damage.

Nevertheless this new model does not constitute no-fault insurance replacing the existing compensation regulations, but complements them: the existing system relies on fault being established.

To date, there is little practical experience of this new compensation-fund system, as most states have just begun to apply it in 2002. The potential advantage is that patients can receive additional compensation, this being a small step in the direction of no-fault insurance.

The weakness lies in the fact that only patients pay into these funds (0.73 Euro per day, 28 days' payment per year maximum): hospitals do not contribute. Furthermore the compensation plans cover public hospitals only, but not doctors working in private practice.

Role and functions

PAs see themselves as:

- the instrument of patients who, for whatever reason, are not able to make themselves understood sufficiently

- a mirror for hospital staff and established doctors, providing external feedback
- an external contributor to safeguarding quality, since they evaluate complaints and hand the results over to healthcare officials
- providing an opportunity to defuse sensitive situations, and create a willingness to enter into discussion
- an extrajudicial institution, to enforce legal claims in an unbureaucratic way, with the corollary of all partners 'saving face'.

Operation

Though employed by states (or in the Tyrol, hospitals), PAs are engaged by patients: they represent patients and act in their interest. There is a wide range of patient-orientated activity, from inquiries, information, and counselling in health and social systems, through complaints based on lack of communication, to implementing solutions in cases of medical malpractice.

The PAs were primarily established in order to provide patients with specialist and qualified representation free of charge. Their effectiveness goes beyond individual casework since PAs can share their experience of processing cases with the authorities responsible and thus instigate preventive measures and structural change. In particular, handling cases of inappropriate or unsuccessful medical treatment offers advantages not only for patients, but also for hospitals and hospital staff concerned. These are:

- quick processing and identification of solutions, bringing conflicts to an end
- no entrenchment of positions
- the likelihood of media sensation is low
- high acceptance, since no legal ramifications and solutions are worked on in agreement with each other.

According to some state laws co-operation with PAs is mandatory for hospitals (they must, for example, provide information and take a position). In this respect, doctors are also obliged to co-operate. Beyond this legal obligation, in practice there is in general well-developed co-operation on a voluntary basis: even though there is no legal obligation for doctors working in practices to co-operate with PAs, co-operation is actually very good in most cases.

Working procedures

Working procedures of PAs vary, but the following procedures are basically the same.

- For inquiries or requests for information which are not actual complaints (for instance inquiries concerning patients' rights), counselling is offered and the patient is at least directed to the appropriate authority.
- General complaints are dealt with in partnership with the patient; the authorities responsible are confronted and asked to take a position. Here, conflicts that have arisen may potentially be resolved or at least moderated. It must be stressed

that this is not an attempt to bring out the objective truth and administer justice, but to make the subjective view of a patient in a certain situation understood by the parties responsible. This feedback, elaborated by PAs, is intended to help develop awareness and inform future patterns of patient-orientated behaviour by interested authorities. This involves patient perceptions in respect of relationships, human treatment, dignity, and so on.

- Where patients present a complaint which involves medical malpractice, legal and medical examinations are carried out (including experts' reports):
  - if for legal and medical reasons malpractice can be ruled out, the patient will be comprehensively informed and counselled (e.g. complications, with an accompanying explanation). Often these complaints are simply based on lack of communication and information, so that a detailed legal and medical explanation takes care of the complaint. The common insecurity of patients which often causes suspicion of malpractice can be cleared in this way
  - complaints with clear fault and sufficient evidence can often be settled by direct negotiation with liability insurance providers. PAs provide the preparatory work necessary for completing a settlement (e.g. a compensation declaration). Compensation law regulations are fully applied and the patient can avail himself of his or her rights with little time invested and no financial risk
  - if there is no possibility of a direct solution with the liability insurance fund (for instance, because of disagreement over fault), or the judgement of medical malpractice is equivocal, arbitration boards are used by the patient. These arbitration boards are either established by the states or by the general medical council (in Vorarlberg, institutions of the state; in Carinthia and Salzburg, part of the PA directly). Arbitration boards draw up a recommended settlement (a judgement of the case by cause and the amount of the compensation payment), but often further hearings will be carried out by PAs (because of additional financial expenses, loss of income, need for nursing care, etc, as a result of malpractice). Neither the patient nor the hospital (liability insurance fund) are bound by these recommendations. The patient always has the option to go to court, if she/he does not agree with the suggestion. In practical terms this happens in very few cases, so the above mentioned procedures save many cases going to trial.

Data

Unfortunately, there are no comparable data for Austria's active PAs. Each PA provides annual reports on their activities, which include a large amount of data, but these are not presented identically. The ARGE initiated a project in 2002 in order to create a nationally standardised, comparable data bank. This report on Austria overall began in summer 2002 as a pilot project and was fully operational from 1 January 2003. Each state's data will be collected and evaluated in Lower Austria.

The following data should then be available:

- total number of complaints over the years (trend data)
- breakdown by institution (hospitals, nursing homes, doctors' surgeries, social insurances, other)
- number of complaints passed on to the mediation agencies of the medical councils

- number of complaints settled with the legal liability insurer directly
- number of cases of malpractice
- quantum of compensation (the total amount of compensation the patients received with the help of the ombudsman)
- ranking of the hospitals according to complaints received.

Data for Lower Austria

Lower Austria is, geographically, the largest state, with 1.55 million inhabitants. 27 public hospitals take care of the population, providing approximately 8000 hospital beds. 2600 doctors working in practice (general practitioners, specialists, dentists) provide further healthcare for the population. By comparison, the smallest state is Vorarlberg, with 370 000 inhabitants, 7 public hospitals, 2166 beds and 300 doctors working in practice.

In 1999–2000 there was a clearly visible increase of 46% in complaints. In 2000–2001 there was a further increase of 10% and in 2001–2002, 25% (*see* Figure 1.1). However this is not seen as an indication that quality is falling in Austria's health and social systems. On the contrary, by way of carefully directed information policies and publicity work the PA has become better known by patients, people who permanently live in institutions, and their relatives. There is a general social trend of increased awareness among the population in terms of their interests, needs and the management of complaints. It is estimated that approximately 50% of complaints are handled by the PAs.

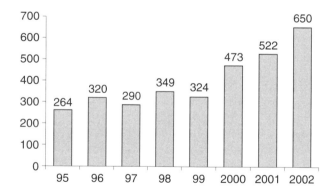

Figure 1.1 Trend in incidence of complaints in Lower Austria, 1995–2002.

It is also extremely important that experience from these complaints is reported back to the institutions concerned. This happens by way of regular lectures in hospitals and nursing homes, by publishing brochures and articles and through a monthly letter on the internet homepage of the Lower Austria PA ('Help Patients').

Differences in complaint frequency in some selected hospitals

Figure 1.2 (below) shows the hospital of 'Sch' receiving one complaint for every 3200 patients; the hospital of 'Mö', one complaint every 500 patients. This means, of course, that the PA of Lower Austria is dealing with many more complaints from the hospital of 'Mö' than from the hospital of 'Sch'.

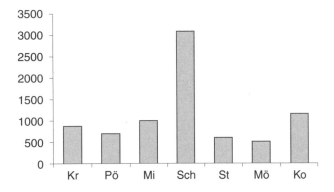

Figure 1.2   Frequency of complaints in selected hospitals in Lower Austria.

These data from hospitals in Lower Austria do not necessarily link to the work of the PAs but do give an indication of whether the complaint management system in the hospital works effectively or not. If it is effective, then fewer complaints tend to reach the PA of Lower Austria.

Analysis and conclusions

The strength of the current system lies in the following points:

- the legal basis and therefore legal legitimacy for PA activities
- independence from hospitals and freedom from direction or influence
- financial security
- general social recognition.

Legal basis

The underpinning law offers a strong formal basis for the PA and with that a classification of the PA as a part of the state. The existence, the tasks and competencies of the PAs are therefore recognised accordingly by the state. Formal classification helps to enforce patients' interests against hospitals and doctors, and the job performed by PAs, being legally defined, needs no further explanation for the parties concerned. The PAs' tasks and activities become integral to the health service and are therefore not seen as interference by a private organisation.

Independence

The independence and freedom from any external direction ensure safety for patients and credibility for PAs. To be a part of the health service (as above) is on the one hand helpful; on the other hand PAs could be suspected of complicity with hospitals. Formal independence therefore gives patients the necessary reassurance. The experiences of the PAs have proved that the independence exists not only 'on paper', but that the political authorities are in practice strictly safeguarding the PAs' independence.

Financial security

The PAs have guaranteed income to carry out their daily work. This comes from the public sector, and therefore there is no dependence on private sponsorship.

General social recognition

The experience of PAs since their introduction has proved their worth; and the public is making use of the services of the PAs more and more. The PAs offer an effective and generally appreciated complaints management system and are invited as a matter of course to input as experts in political decision making. The PAs have the opportunity to present their work in many healthcare environments and to offer their conclusions and advice.

The ARGE in particular is very well perceived in its operations at federal state level and has the opportunity from time to time to give expert input into deliberations on federal legislation. The ARGE's credibility in this respect is aided by the fact that all PAs are university graduates; most of them are jurists, and they also count a physician and a psychologist among their ranks.

The weaknesses of the system lie in the following areas:

- differences in competencies
- differences in structures
- the appointment of a PA is limited to five years in most states (except Lower Austria, where the appointment is for an unlimited period).

Differences in competencies

The variations in competencies of the PAs from state to state are very restrictive for the patients. Often patients may have received treatment in both hospital and a doctor's surgery, but some PAs can only investigate one aspect of this. For patients it is also difficult to understand why PAs may investigate treatment in hospital but not in the doctor's surgery. This chapter suggests that an expansion of the competencies in all states is necessary.

Differences in structures

A centralised model for a PA covering a state in its entirety has proven effective, since a collective knowledge of all health facilities in the state can be built up. Treatment in several hospitals can therefore be effectively checked by one institution. This model should be replicated across all the federal states of Austria.

However, this centralised organisation also has disadvantages, particularly for the larger states. Sometimes the patients may need to travel large distances to get to the PA, which is often far removed from the daily work of the hospital. The solution to this would be to establish specialist Ombudsmen in all hospitals. These operate in hospitals as a first port of call; if they cannot reach a solution (i.e. the patient is dissatisfied), the patient should then be able to submit their case to the PA. However, it should be possible in any event to go directly to the PA as well; in cases of malpractice, the PA should be given exclusive competency.

The PA would need to keep in touch with the local Ombudsmen, support their work and provide further education. In Lower Austria a pilot project is planned to look at creating an 'Ombudsman network'.

Limited duration of appointment

Independence is very important but creates risks, because of the limited period of the appointment of most of the PAs. So, if a PA creates too many difficulties for the health service, they run the risk of not having their contract renewed by the political authorities. The situation therefore calls for permanent appointment of all PAs (as is the case in Lower Austria); this might be preceded by an appointment period of about five years to establish whether or not the PA is appropriate and fit for permanent appointment. Subsequently, appointments need to be permanent (mirroring the appointment of judges in Austria).

Evaluation

At present, there is no structured and planned evaluation being carried out on the PA system. Without doubt this would be an extremely important piece of work and a proposal for this will be discussed in the ARGE in 2003.

CHAPTER 2

The Ombudsman in Finland

Lars Fallberg and Mervi Kattelus

Introduction

The Finnish healthcare system has a number of similarities with the system in Sweden owing to the history shared by the two countries. But instead of organising health services into counties (as is the case in Sweden), in Finland municipalities are responsible for organizing healthcare for their citizens. The population of a municipality varies from less than 1000 inhabitants to about 500 000, the average being about 11 000.

Two legal acts play an important role in protecting the rights of Finnish patients. Following the Swedish voluntary No-Fault Patient Compensation Scheme, the Finnish Patient Injuries Act was introduced in 1986 (585/1986). The aim of the law was to improve the legal status of patients and define what type of treatment-related events may lead to financial compensation. In 1992, having debated issues of patients' rights for nearly 20 years, the Act on the Status and Rights of Patients (785/1992) was finally passed by the Finnish Parliament. The Finnish law on patients' rights, claimed to be the first in the world, regulates the principles central to patient care and treatment. It also has a section introducing the Patient Ombudsman institution and its role and function in Finnish health services.

The Patient Injuries Act

One aim of introducing the Patient Injuries Act was that it was regarded as more appropriate to solve issues related to patient injuries between the patient and an insurer instead of through a tort claim against the doctor and the healthcare institution. Today all Finnish healthcare providers, public and private, are required to participate in the patient insurance scheme. Seven categories of incident, ranging from maltreatment to psychological effects of the maltreatment, are compensated by the insurance. All claims are sent to the Finnish Patient Insurance Center (FPIC), which reviews all cases free of charge to the complainant. The compensation paid by the insurance company as a member of the FPIC is not dependent on the negligence of healthcare staff. Only if healthcare staff have injured a patient deliberately or through gross negligence will the insurer have the right to recourse against them. If patients are not satisfied with the review made by the

FPIC they have the opportunity to ask an opinion from the Patient Injuries Board (PIB). The PIB does not have the authority to change the decision taken by the FPIC, but its recommendation is highly respected by the FPIC.

The Act on the Status and Rights of Patients

The Finnish Act on Patients' Rights entered into force on 1 March 1993. The aim of the law was not to create an exhaustive list of all possible patients' rights. Instead, central principles of patients' rights were codified in order to clarify and strengthen those rights. Being labelled a 'law of rights', the Finnish law is mainly built on the obligations of healthcare staff or authorities.

The principal contents of the Act are:

- the right to care (section 3)
- access to treatment (section 4)
- the right to information (section 5)
- the right to self-determination (section 6)
- the status of minor patients (section 7)
- emergency treatment (section 8)
- the right to representation (section 9)
- complaints (section 10)
- Patient Ombudsman (section 11)
- medical documentation (section 12)
- confidentiality (section 13).

Patients' 'right to care' embraces individuals who live permanently in the country but has a very important limitation, namely the availability of resources.

> Every person who stays in Finland permanently, is without discrim-
> ination, entitled to the health and medical care required by his state of
> health within the limits of those resources which are available to the
> healthcare at the time in question (§ 1).

Recent jurisprudence of the Finnish Supreme Administrative Court shows, however, that lack of resources cannot be the sole reason for refusing treatment or, for
example, medical appliances, from the patient.

The Act does not require patients' written consent to care and treatment. Instead,
the wording is softer: the patient has to be cared for in mutual understanding with
him/her. In practice, the patient's explicit consent is not asked for every minor
treatment or measure but if the patient refuses a certain treatment or measure, the
healthcare staff have to find another medically acceptable way to treat him/her.
There is a specific provision concerning consent of a minor (persons under 18 years
of age). A proposal to set the limit at 12 was discussed, but the provision was left
more flexible:

> The opinion of a minor patient on a given treatment has to be assessed
> if this is possible with regard to his/her age or level of development.

The law also requires every care unit to have a special Patient Ombudsman. The tasks of this official under the Act are described further in the text.

Organisational structure

The Act provides that every healthcare unit in Finland, public and private, is obliged to appoint a Patient Ombudsman. Following this provision, today more than 2000 Patient Ombudsmen are in post locally across Finland. As it is the Finnish municipalities which have the financial and organisational responsibility for public healthcare services, it is they who act as the principal or employer of the Patient Ombudsman. Most Patient Ombudsmen are, however, appointed by private health-care units; e.g. in the northern region of Lapland, according to one survey, 30% of Ombudsmen worked in the public sector, and 65% in the private sector. The reason for these unbalanced figures is that in Finland in general there are more private healthcare units than public. However, these private units are small, and they provide only a fraction of the healthcare services in total because the public system is the main system in Finland. Owing to the decentralised responsibility of organising and managing the Patient Ombudsmen, in practice the position and function can be subject to local independent agreement between the Ombudsman and the healthcare unit or the municipality.

A Patient Ombudsman may share his/her (most often her) work between two or more healthcare units. When someone is appointed to work as a Patient Ombudsman, this task is normally carried out in addition to his or her regular function as a social worker or nurse. This situation has raised the issue between Patient Ombudsmen themselves as to whether they should be disqualified, from time to time, from dealing with certain matters. There are, however, few Ombudsmen working within a large hospital or responsible for several units at the same time. When this is the case, the Ombudsman works full time without having to share his/her time with other duties.

As mentioned earlier, Patient Ombudsmen are mainly recruited from social workers or nurses at the local health unit. There are no requirements as to any specific education or special training needed to become an Ombudsman. Surveys of the Patient Ombudsman system show that sometimes Ombudsmen are appointed haphazardly and without any minimum requirements and, because of their other tasks, they are unable to concentrate on their job as a Patient Ombudsman. In recent years, however, the number of Ombudsmen with some legal training has increased.

Provincial governments, the National Authority for Medico-Legal Affairs, local governments, universities, patients' organisations etc organise the practical and theoretical training of Ombudsmen. All training and education are arranged on a voluntary basis and depend on the approval of the employer of the Patient Ombudsman to let him or her participate.

There is still no uniform, national training for Ombudsmen. Several organisations and institutes provide information and training. A working group of the Provincial Board of Southern Finland proposed in February 2002 that there should be a national working group, whose task would be to plan the content of this training and possibly to start it in further education centres of universities. However, this proposal has not yet been realised.

Role and functions

One of the key features of the Finnish law on patients' rights is the introduction of the Patient Ombudsman institution. The law provides that the tasks of Patient Ombudsmen are the following:

- to advise patients in issues concerning the application of the act
- to help patients in the matters covered in paragraphs 1 and 3 of section 10 (complaints and liability questions)
- to inform patients of their rights
- to act also otherwise for the promotion and implementation of patients' rights.

The task of the Patient Ombudsman is largely to inform and advise patients and citizens about the existence and content of the patients' rights law. The idea is that providing information will influence attitudes, prevent conflicts and, as a final result, promote patients' rights.

Operation

Patients may, at any given time, approach or contact the Ombudsman to get information or to launch a complaint. Information on how to get in contact with the Patient Ombudsman is normally available at the healthcare unit or other healthcare facilities, and can also be found from the website of many municipalities. A recent study, however, shows that information on Patient Ombudsmen is not always easily, or even at all, available.

The role of the Finnish Ombudsman is not, under any circumstances, to become the representative or 'Ombud' of the patient. The Ombud is an employee of the healthcare unit but shall act as independently as possible in relation to both healthcare staff and to the patients and/or complainants. In addition to providing information about the patients' rights law, the Ombud has the duty to receive complaints from patients and their family and friends and to make informal investigations based upon the complaint.

It is important to emphasise that the Finnish Patient Ombudsman does not have any rights or powers to decide on sanctions or make official recommendations. The Ombudsman may not assist patients in the event of a trial in court and does not have any independent right to make decisions within the health unit.

Statistical information

There are no national statistics on the number or the nature of cases handled by Patient Ombudsmen. This is partly owing to the very decentralised nature of the Patient Ombudsman system. In addition, there is no legal obligation for Patient Ombudsmen to keep records, collect statistics, or analyse developments and trends of the cases they handle.

Several local surveys of the system have, however, been made. The information given here is mainly based on the survey made by the Provincial Board of Lapland (*Patient Ombudsman Activities in the Province of Lapland – Year 2001*). A survey in

2001 was carried out by a questionnaire that was sent to 102 Patient Ombudsmen in that region. Out of these 62% replied to the questionnaire. Most Patient Ombudsmen had healthcare education (71%), the next largest group (19%) had some form of social welfare education, and the rest (10%) some other education. More than 61% had over four years of experience of these tasks and 25% had been working as Patient Ombudsmen for 7–10 years. More than half of them had participated in training given to Patient Ombudsmen, but 37% had not received any form of training.

Out of those who answered the questionnaire, 65% spent less than one hour a week on Patient Ombudsman tasks. A quarter spent one to two hours a week and only 5% over seven hours a week on these tasks. Most Patient Ombudsmen (92%) did not get any compensation for their work.

The number of patient contacts varies considerably. In this survey 61% had less than two contacts per year and 20% had two to ten contacts per year. One Patient Ombudsman had 100 contacts and another one more than 200 contacts per year. According to another survey in Southern Finland (*Patient Empowerment*, Provincial Board of Southern Finland, 2002), where the units are generally bigger, the number of patient contacts have been several hundred or even more than a thousand per year.

In Lapland, patients asked most frequently (57%) about their treatment and/or medical examination. In 40% of the cases the reason for contact was inappropriate behaviour or treatment by healthcare personnel. Problems concerning lack of information were also a general reason (14%) for contacts. Most contacts (48%) concerned medical doctors.

Patients' contacts with Patient Ombudsmen led to their giving advice to the patient in 49% of the cases, to patient insurance claims in 43% and to complaints within the healthcare unit in question in 27% of the cases.

Analysis

Finland's introduction of Patient Ombudsmen into the healthcare sector came at the end of a long period of debate about patients' rights. The Patient Ombudsman, by some people regarded as the patients' ambassador, created expectations among patients and citizens. The intention was that the relationship between patients and healthcare staff would become a more equal one. These expectations were created not just by the way every Finnish health unit was obliged to appoint a Patient Ombudsman; in addition, using the term 'Ombudsman' ('*Potilasasiamies*' in Finnish) implied that someone was appointed, by law, to speak and act on behalf of patients who are in a condition where it is difficult to protect their own rights.

This very positive image of the Patient Ombudsman was presented not only to citizens residing in Finland, but also to neighbouring countries. The general opinion was that by introducing the new law on patients' rights and the provision on Patient Ombudsmen, Finland had taken a very important step towards democracy in the health services and patient empowerment.

However, analysing the law and how it has been implemented, it would not be an exaggeration to say that the law on patients' rights is rather weak and the provision of Patient Ombudsmen creates a somewhat false sense of protection and safety for patients. It is true that the implementation process emphasised some areas more than others. Nevertheless, the patients' rights law has several weaknesses as regards the Ombudsman system. Some are more pertinent than others.

- A majority of all Patient Ombudsmen have regular positions as social workers or nurses at the same unit. There is an obvious risk for conflict of interest.
- Patient Ombudsmen have the same employer as the healthcare staff who may be the subject of the conflict with the complainant. Here, also, there is an obvious risk of conflict of interest.
- There are no formal requirements as to what kind of training or education is required to become a Patient Ombudsman.
- When first introduced, there was a lack of co-ordination between the Ombudsmen regarding e.g. statistics, training and sharing experiences. However, this has gradually improved.
- The official name 'Patient Ombudsman' implies that the institution in some way represents and/or acts on behalf of patients. However, the Patient Ombudsman is strictly a provider of information and guidance within the system.

In a recent analysis of the Patient Ombudsman system it is pointed out that the system does not work as it was meant to in the act. The most pertinent problems at this time are:

- lack of or insufficient knowledge and education among the Ombudsmen
- dependent position as one of the employees of the healthcare unit
- insufficient resources and underestimation of the importance of their tasks.

Conclusions

The Finnish patients' rights law is now 10 years old. It has become well known across Europe and is in some countries regarded as a model law emphasising the Patient Ombudsman institution. However, the law lacks teeth and does not necessarily give individual patients sufficient legal protection in the case of a conflict. All of the 'rights' provided in the law are conditioned by the availability of resources or lack a sufficiently precise definition to stand up in court. Nevertheless, recent court cases indicate that lack of resources is not a good enough reason for health authorities to refuse patients their rights according to the law. The implementation of the patients' rights law was expected to be carried out by the Patient Ombudsmen. Taking into account the lack of preparation and training given to the Patient Ombudsmen when the law was introduced in 1993 it is both surprising and encouraging to see how quickly they adapted to the situation and formed networks among themselves.

It is unclear what the effect of the Ombudsman provision has been in terms of knowledge about the content of the patients' rights law among patients, patients' families and healthcare staff. There seems to be no scientific research on the supposed increased level of understanding about patients' rights among Finnish citizens.

It is probably true to say that the Finnish law on patients' rights was a signal from the legislature of the need for increased effort to strengthen the role of patients in Finnish health services. The law itself, however, is not always enough to support someone who would like to demand his/her rights in court. The Patient Ombudsman provision should be discussed in connection with legal reforms related to the patients' rights law. If the task of the Patient Ombudsman is to continue to be one of information provider, then consideration could be given to changing its name to 'Patient Guide' or 'Patient Adviser'. To name the institution according to its real function would probably be a positive step in the long run, in that it will begin to rebuild a relationship of trust between patients and citizens on the one hand, and the authorities on the other. In any case it is necessary to emphasise the independence, formal training and power of the Ombudsman.

Further reading

* Etelä-Suomen lääninhallitus: Potilaan aseman vahvistaminen (Patient Empowerment, Working Group Report) (2002) *Terveydenhuolto 2000-luvulle-projektin osaraportti.*
* Eyben B (ed.) (2001) *Alternative Compensation Mechanisms for Damages.* Dansk Selskab for Forsikringsret (Danish Section of the International Association for Insurance Law), Copenhagen.
* Fallberg L (2000) Patients' rights in the Nordic countries. *Eur J Health Law.* **6**: 123–43.
* Fallberg L (2001) Patients' rights in Europe: where do we stand and where do we go? *Eur J Health Law.* **7**: 1–3.
* Hannikainen P *et al.* (1996) Three years in force: has the Finnish act on the status and rights of patients materialized? Report from the Finnish Ministry of Health and Social Affairs. *Sosiaali- ja terveysministeriön monisteita.* **4**.
* Kestilä M (2001) Potilasasiamiestoiminta Lapin läänissä vuonna (Patient Ombudsman Activities in the Province of Lapland – Year 2001). *Lapin lääninhallituksen julkaisusarja.* **7**.
* Koivuniemi P (1994) Potilasasiamiestiminnalle on määriteltävä vaatimustaso (A standard has to be defined for patient ombudsman functions). *J Finnish Med Assoc.* **49**: 2704–05.
* Kokkonen P (1994) The new Finnish law on the status and rights of a patient. *Eur J Health Law.* **1**: 127–36.
* Lahti R (1994) Towards a comprehensive legislation governing the rights of patients: the Finnish experience. In: L Westerhäll and C Phillips (eds) *Patients' Rights – informed consent, access and equality.* Nerenius & Santérus Publishers, Göteborg, pp. 207–21.
* Modeen T (1994) *Patienten I hälso- och sjukvården.* Juristförbundets förlag, Helsinki.

CHAPTER 3

The Greek Ombudsman and the protection of patients' rights

Eftichis Fitrakis and Ioanna Arsenopoulou

Introduction*

The geopolitical position and the constitutional framework in Greece

Greece is situated in south-east Europe and covers an area of approximately 132 000 km², most of which is mountainous or islands. It has approximately 11 million inhabitants.** The country has been a member of the European Union since 1981 and participates in the monetary union and the Western European Union. It is also a member of NATO and a member of the major supranational institutions for the protection of democratic principles and human rights, such as the Council of Europe.

The Greek system of government is a parliamentary democracy. During the 20th century the country's system of government was modified on numerous occasions. This was owing to the fluidity of the political situation after the two world wars and the cold war, which prevailed until the end of the 1960s.[1,2] Furthermore, the imposition and the collapse of the military dictatorship in the years between 1967 and 1974 led to the abolition of the monarchy and, in the end, with the constitution of 1975, to the establishment of parliamentary democracy.[3,4] In accordance with Article 26 of the constitution, 'Legislative power shall be vested in Parliament and the President of the Republic'; 'Executive power shall be vested in the President of the Republic and the Government', while 'Judicial power shall be vested in the courts of law …'.

---

* Dr E Fitrakis is the author of Chapter 3 to p. 47 and Dr I Arsenopoulou the author of the rest of the Chapter.
** In accordance with data from the recent (2001) census, the exact population of Greece is 10 939 605.

The status and role of public administration

Public administration in Greece is comprised of the public sector services and the public corporate agencies. Public administration is the medium through which executive power is realised. For this reason, the public administration is accountable to the government, whose political decisions are responsible for implementing it. It should be noted that, while members of the government set the political direction, civil servants are committed to follow the principle of neutrality, or, more specifically, are obliged to be politically impartial. Traditionally, the functions of the public administration are distinguished in three categories:

- a restrictive function (this includes control services, such as maintaining order, collection of taxes, etc)
- a function for providing services (e.g. social insurance, health and social-welfare services, etc)
- a regulatory function (e.g. programming, guidelines, etc).

The Greek state was established after the 1821 war of independence. Administratively it was essentially organised by the Bavarian staff of King Othon (1832 and after). The organisation of public administration was based on foreign standards, which, very often, were simply translated and became laws of the Greek state. This importation of foreign models without the necessary tailoring to suit the Greek cultural and political background, instead of facilitating the smooth operation of the administrative machine to solve existing problems, complicated the situation and hindered efforts to find solutions.

The administrative problem

The gradual expansion of the state was linked to widening democracy. State intervention in social and economic development was accompanied by a replacement of the, until then, 'restrictive' police state with the welfare state.[5] Thus, the expansion of state activities led to a tremendous growth of the public administrative machine and to the economic position which results from such growth. Consequently, maladministration, to a certain degree, is linked to the huge size of the civil service.

   The problems that the Greek public administration presents relate to both the structural level, including manpower, and to the operational level.[6] Moreover, the intense politicisation of the public administration has had a serious detrimental influence on its effectiveness. These matters contribute to the crisis of legitimacy of the public administration. Civil servants often act arbitrarily, violating the rule of law. Thus, in the context of the need for modernisation of the public administration, two problems must be dealt with: its legitimacy and its effectiveness.

The need for the institution of the Ombudsman

The development of the post-war Greek state was closely linked to a series of human rights violations, especially during the period of the cold war. Discrimination, policies of exclusion and arbitrary decision-making were characteristic of the administrative apparatus, sometimes representing state policy. Thus, the public administration often failed to perform its function of serving the citizen and became instead oppressive to the people. This traditional form of public administration generated the need for the development of mechanisms which would effectively protect the individual from arbitrary administrative decisions. The advance of traditionally less favoured socio-economic powers progressively led to the creation of a system of guarantees and protection mechanisms for the support of human rights. On that basis, the protection of citizens' rights, beyond the basic acknowledgement of their existence, relied on the provision of a series of supervisory procedures.

In Greek law, traditionally, three different types of control were provided for the public administration.[7,8]

1 Parliamentary control of the government, which constitutes a very significant parliamentary activity. This type of supervision by its nature has, to a certain extent, political implications as it is linked to the balance between political parties in Parliament.
2 Judicial review, which constitutes the most classical form of control of the public administration in a state operating with respect for the rule of law. This type of control is carried out through a system of administrative justice, at the top of which is the 'Council of State'.
3 Administrative self-control, which is exercised in terms of:
   – hierarchical control
   – formal petitions
   – administrative supervision
   – financial control, or finally
   – inspections by 'The Public Administration Investigators–Inspectors Authority'.

In the last few decades it has been consistently shown that these traditional ways of administrative control do not meet the real requirements of a modern liberal society, which is centred on the principle of respect for the rights of its citizens. The failure of the existing control mechanisms to adequately respond to the demand for full supervision of the relations between the citizen and the state generated the need to identify new forms of institutions to fill the void.

'O Synigoros tou Politi' (citizen's advocate) or, as it is best known internationally, the Ombudsman, is such an institution. In the Greek scheme of things the Ombudsman constitutes a fourth level of administrative control. The Ombudsman operates alongside the other existing institutions, exercising control over public administration, without replacing them. Its jurisdiction covers, furthermore, areas of maladministration that do not fall within the jurisdiction of the three other types of institutional control, and has certain options for action not available to those others.

The system of protection of patients' rights

In Greece, both the public and private sectors provide health services. The overwhelming majority of these services are provided by the public sector. Private clinics, hospitals, outpatient health facilities and laboratories provide only a small part of the health service in Greece. There is no intensive administrative scrutiny whatsoever of health service provision by the private sector. Nevertheless, private health units are under the supervision of local government departments.

The public system of health includes hospitals, health centres and outpatient facilities. These belong to the state or to the public insurance funds. Organisationally and hierarchically these services fall within the fabric of state administration and are organised as sub-sectors of public administration. Thus, the relationship with a patient-user of health services, in whichever (public) health unit, is one of state–citizen or, better, it is a relation between the one who administers and the citizen. A person's visit to a health facility can be seen as a citizen versus state issue, though the state here consists of a single health unit. As a result, the inspection of a (public) health unit involves all three aforementioned traditional forms of control, i.e. parliamentary, judicial and administrative self-control.

The progressive elevation of patients' rights in social debate and the realisation of the need for patients' protection led to the strengthening of administrative self-control mechanisms in all public health units. Thus, it was legislated that every hospital should have a three-member 'Committee for the Defence of Patients' Rights' (Article 1, para 4, of Act 2519/1997).[9] Simultaneously, in the Ministry of Health and Social Welfare two committees were set up: the 'Independent Service for the Protection of Patients' Rights', which directly answers to the general secretary of the Ministry, and the 'Control Committee for the Protection of Patients' Rights'. In addition, in the Ministry of Health and Social Welfare, another committee named 'Ad Hoc Committee for the Rights of the Individuals with Psychical Disorders' was established. Its membership comprises those with acknowledged expertise on the subject. Furthermore, the 'Office for the Protection of Persons with Psychological Disorders' was also created (Article 2, para 1, of Act 2716/1999). This committee answers directly to the Minister of Health and Social Welfare, that is, it does not belong to the established administrative hierarchy.

Nevertheless, the operation of current administrative self-regulation does not appear to have produced satisfactory results, for two main reasons:

- the absence of independence for these control mechanisms. Usually the person who investigates is subordinate to the person being investigated
- the lack of essential will to support these statutory control mechanisms.

Thus, not only in terms of staffing but also in terms of technical infrastructure no real efforts were made to realise the original legislative aim. It did, however, remain a wish for some individuals alive to the problem, given that the existing system was not able to instigate real institutional change.

To remedy this, in accordance with Act 2920/2001, 'The Public Administration Investigators of Health and Welfare Services' was recently established. This particular service, which comes under the remit of the Minister of Heath, has as its purpose the systematic inspection of healthcare services. The main objective of The Public Administration Investigators of Health and Welfare Services is to increase quality and eliminate maladministration in health services.[10]

Brief historical background

Greece has one independent mediating authority, that is, it has a single Ombudsman institution. Its jurisdiction extends over public sector services in their entirety. Thus in Greece, in contrast with other countries, there are no separate Ombudsmen overseeing particular areas of the public sector, for example, of health, of the military forces, of children's services, etc. Therefore, maladministration issues in health, in the absence of a Health Ombudsman as a separate institution, fall within the jurisdiction of the (general) Ombudsman. However, with the introduction of Act 3094/2003, issues concerning the welfare of children will be examined by a separate department named 'Children's Rights Protection Department'.

The establishment of the Greek Ombudsman as an independent authority, in accordance with Act 2477/97 (now Act 3094/2003), marks the culmination of a long struggle to improve the public sector and its relations with the citizen. It is important to note that this legislation had the unanimous support of all political parties. The few reservations that were expressed focused on the issue of strengthening the powers and the areas of jurisdiction of the Ombudsman and were not a criticism of the need for its existence. In any case, there was unanimity regarding the need for genuine and independent control of the public administration for the sake of the protection of citizens' rights.

The creation of the Greek institution of the Ombudsman took into consideration the respective models of other European countries, but it essentially followed its own distinctive pattern. It is important to note that both major political parties (the government and the opposition) had tabled earlier drafts of the law for the establishment of the Ombudsman in Parliament in 1995–96. The final draft, which later became Act 2477/97, contained many of the elements included in the earlier drafts. Of course this issue was already the object of debate by administrative scientists and experts in administrative law. In January 2003 a new law was introduced (Act 3094/2003) which transformed and amended the existing law (Act 2477/97).

At an earlier stage, however, considerable effort had been put into the issue of controlling maladministration through the establishment of 'The Public Administration Investigators–Inspectors Authority', which was a semi-independent, many-member body that functioned within the public administration.[11] That body essentially operated from 1990 and was completely renewed with the establishment of the Ombudsman. The prevailing view was that this earlier institution constituted the transitional stage towards the consolidation of a truly external mechanism of control of public administration and for mediation between the citizen and the state.

The constitutional revision of 2001 safeguarded the institution of the Ombudsman as an independent authority.[12] A law defines the issues pertinent to the formation and the jurisdictions of the Greek Ombudsman, which functions as an independent authority. Relevant to the function of the Ombudsman are the provisions of the revised constitution concerning independent authorities. (*See* Article 101A of the constitution.)

- Wherever the constitution envisages the establishment and operation of an independent authority, its members are appointed for a specified period of duty and are bound to exercise personal and operational independence, as the law provides.
- A law provides for issues pertinent to the selection and the service status of scientific and other personnel in the public service, who are appointed to

support the operation of each independent authority. Their selection is made according to the ruling of the board of Parliament chairmen, with unanimity if possible, or otherwise with a majority vote of four-fifths of its members. A parliamentary regulation governs the selection procedure.

- The parliamentary regulation regulates the relationship between Parliament and the independent authorities as well as the system of parliamentary control.

The motion for this constitutional change again had the unanimous support of all political parties represented in Parliament. This constitutional platform for the Ombudsman contributed substantially to its prestige and further strengthens its institutional independence. As a result, it is no longer possible for the general legislature to abolish or substantially change the nature or the role of the Ombudsman. Furthermore, with this constitutional safeguard the institution of the Ombudsman becomes an inseparable and stable part of the state, as opposed to a temporary result of political decisions. In May 1998 the first Ombudsman was selected, and by October of the same year the institution began functioning fully with the receipt of citizens' complaints.

The approval of citizens and the civil service, as well as the support of the mass media, were among the basic elements which, from the outset, were considered necessary for the success of the Ombudsman.[13] For the Greek Ombudsman its legitimacy and acceptance as an impartial institution and a mechanism for the strict application of the law was a major objective. It is true that the establishment of the Ombudsman received the approval and the support, but also embodied the hopes and expectations, of both citizens and the political sectors. Three years after the establishment of the authority, it appears to have won, to a considerable degree, the respect and the approval of citizens as an independent authority for the protection and consolidation of the rule of law. Criticisms that are sometimes made focus on the Ombudsman's lack of decision-making powers that would permit some control over public administrators. The mass media often make reference to the work of the authority, and to a very high degree have a positive attitude towards the institution and its work. Nevertheless, it must be pointed out that, while this positive attitude contributes to the legitimacy of the authority in the eyes of the public, it simultaneously raises expectations that cannot always be fulfilled.

Organisational structure

Position

In accordance with Article 101, para 1 of the constitution, 'The administration of the state shall be organised on the basis of decentralisation'. This way, enough latitude is provided for the regional state bodies to make decisions while the 'central organs of the state shall have, in addition to special authorities, the general guidance, co-ordination and the supervision of the actions of the regional functionaries'. In parallel with this, in Greece there is in effect a system of first and second tiers of local government. In accordance with Article 102, para 1 of the constitution 'the administration of local affairs shall be exercised by the first and second tiers of the local government agencies'.

The Ombudsman in Greece operates centrally with a service unit based in Athens. Issues of decentralisation and the establishment of regional offices by law are still being planned at this stage. From time to time though a team of experts from the authority visits certain provincial cities (capitals of regions) and at least once a year a visit is made to Thessaloniki, the second largest city in the country. The jurisdiction of the Ombudsman covers every public service in the country, irrespective of whether it is a part of central or local government. Thus, every public sector service at the level of municipality, prefecture, region or the ministry is included in its jurisdiction.

Funding

The issue of funding for the institution is very important because its independence and its ability to reach its aims depend on it. The Ombudsman as a public authority is exclusively funded by government. The funds needed for the operation of the Ombudsman are entered in a special account and incorporated in the annual budget of the Ministry of Interior, Public Administration and Decentralisation (Article 1 of the Act 3094/2003).

Internal organisation

The work of the authority is organised in the following four departments:*

1 Department of Human Rights
2 Department of Health and Social Welfare (social policy, health, insurance, welfare of children, elderly and people with special needs)
3 Department of the Quality of Life (environment, urban planning, land use, public works, culture)
4 Department of State–Citizen Relations (information and communication, quality of services provided, maladministration in local administration and public utility companies, transportation, communication, work, industry, energy, taxation, customs, financial issues, trade and state provisions, agriculture and agricultural policy, education).

With the introduction of Act 3094/2003 a new department has been established, exclusively for the protection of children's rights.

Professional staff

According to the institution's founding law, the Ombudsman is assisted in carrying out his duties by four Deputy Ombudsmen. In addition to the Ombudsman and the Deputy Ombudsmen, senior and junior investigators

---

* The internal organisation of the authority is governed by Presidential Decree 273/1999 [Regulations of the Ombudsman].

support the work of the office. By the end of 2001, 77 individuals had joined the staff, 23 of them seconded from other civil service posts and 54 newly recruited. Of these 77 individuals, 49 joined as senior investigators and 28 as junior investigators. During 2001 an administrative staff of 28 people were employed at the office of the Ombudsman. The professional staff of the authority who conduct the investigations covers a wide range of specialities, while 50% of them have legal training.

Accountability

According to the constitution, the Ombudsman is an independent authority. In addition, Article 2, para 1 of Act 3051/2002 stipulates that 'The independent authorities are not subject to supervision by any government body or administrative authority'. However, the Ombudsman is subject to Parliament, where a general account of the work of the institution must be given. Specifically, in accordance with Article 3, para 5 of Act 3094/2003:

> The Ombudsman produces an annual report in which he sets out the work of the authority, presents the most important cases and makes recommendations regarding the improvement of public services and the required legislative regulations. The Ombudsman's report is submitted in March of each year to the chairman of Parliament and the report is discussed during a special plenary session. The report is also published in a special issue by the National Printing Office. The Ombudsman may also submit it to the prime minister, the chairman of the Parliament.

Also every year the Ombudsman appears personally in front of the 'Select Committee on Institutions and Transparency', where Members of Parliament question him about the work of the authority. Finally, it should be noted that the Ombudsman and the Deputy Ombudsmen are not held responsible, prosecuted, or subjected to inquiry for any opinion expressed or action performed during the exercise of their duties (personal immunity of the heads of institutions).

Role and function

Aims and objectives

The Ombudsman in Greece was created for two main reasons:

1 to be a mediator between the state and the citizen
2 to be a commissioner for public administration.

As is stipulated in Article 1, para 1 of Act 3094/2003, the institution was established 'with the aim of protecting the rights of citizens, combating maladministration, and ensuring observance of the law'. In this way the Ombudsman is in the service of the public interest without being linked to either the public administration or the citizen who submits a complaint. The mediating and the supervisory objectives of the Ombudsman are predicated on two basic elements: independence and credibility. A mediator is an individual who, for both parties, remains a 'third' person, without supporting the position of the one or the other. Also, true protection of the rights of citizens must come from decisions and opinions developed only after a careful, systematic investigation of the facts of a case. In avoiding, in principle, any untoward or hasty condemnation of the public administration, the Ombudsman is given greater strength to carry out his/her investigative work.[14]

The Greek Ombudsman has repeatedly declared a firm position in favour of the 'logic of unravelling' problems, at the same time rejecting the 'logic of conflict and denunciation' as a means of settling differences.[15] The Ombudsman also strongly professes the theory of 'positive sum' (all parties can win in a case, to a greater or lesser extent), as compared with the logic of 'zero sum' (one wins, the other must lose).

Terms of reference

The Ombudsman has jurisdiction over issues pertaining to:

- public sector
- first and second tiers of local government
- public corporate bodies
- public companies (Article 3, of the Act 3094/2003).

The Ombudsman does not have any jurisdiction over:

- government ministers and deputy ministers for acts pertaining to their political functions
- religious entities underpinned by public law
- judicial authorities
- military services with regard to issues of national defence and security
- the National Intelligence Service
- services of the Ministry of Foreign Affairs for matters relating to the conduct of the country's foreign policy or international relations
- the Legal Council of the State and independent authorities with regard to their principal functions.

The Ombudsman investigates personal administrative acts or omissions or material acts of public service bodies that violate or infringe the legal interests of physical persons or legal entities. In particular, he investigates cases in which a public service body, individual or collective:

- infringes, by act or omission, a right or interest protected by the constitution and the law
- refuses to fulfil a specific obligation imposed by final judicial judgement
- refuses to fulfil a specific obligation imposed by a legal provision or by a personal administrative act
- performs or omits to perform a legal duty in violation of the principles of transparency and proper administration or in abuse of power.

The Ombudsman cannot investigate cases pending before a judicial authority.

Powers

Investigation of cases

The Ombudsman may ask public sector services to provide him with any information, document or other evidence relating to the case, and may examine individuals, perform an on-site examination and order an expert's report (Article 4 of the Act 3094/2003). These powers of the Ombudsman demonstrate the pre-eminence of the authority and contribute to ensuring an independent and unbiased decision in every particular case.[16] A large caseload is managed with, in each case, relevant documents being forwarded to the Ombudsman by public sector services. Afterwards the Ombudsman may pose certain questions, as necessary, which will help to clarify the facts of the case. Examination of witnesses occurs only when the information provided by an individual (private person or public servant) needs to be corroborated. Lastly, an on-site examination is often carried out in order to determine real events, or circumstances, but it can also occur in order to form an opinion about the workings of a particular civil service. Usually, on-site examinations are undertaken to gain an understanding of the relevant environment, but they can also be performed to uncover how a public service, for example a hospital or another type of institution, works in practice. On-site examinations, by the Ombudsman staff in person and without prior warning, are also performed in order to search the records of certain public sector services. This has occurred in cases involving hospitals where there has been a real danger of falsification or concealment of medical data.

Finally, an expert's report can be commissioned from an external private expert, or other public agencies. The purpose of commissioning an external agent to produce a report is to clarify a serious scientific or technical matter that requires expert knowledge. This power of the Ombudsman has not yet been exercised, mainly because the wide range of specialisation of its own professional staff covers, to a large extent, the necessary expertise to complete the work in hand, without having to resort to external assistance. Such expert investigation is first and foremost useful in the investigation especially of cases which involve issues of medical malpractice.[17]

Completion of the investigation

On completion of the investigation, the Ombudsman draws up a report on the findings, to be communicated to the competent minister and authorities, and mediates as far as possible to resolve the citizen's problem. In his recommendations to public sector services, the Ombudsman must set a time limit within which those services have an obligation to inform him of action taken to implement his recommendations, or of the reasons for which they cannot accept them. The Ombudsman may make a refusal to accept recommendations public, if he considers that this is not sufficiently justified. If there is sufficient evidence that a public sector employee, civil servant, or member of an administration has committed a criminal act, the Ombudsman must also communicate the report to the competent public prosecutor.

Operation

The right of petition and the form of complaint

Article 10, para 1 of the (Greek) constitution states that 'Each person, acting on their own or together with others, shall have the right … to petition in writing public authorities, who shall be obliged to respond promptly in accordance with the provisions in force, and to justify their answers …'. Thus the 'right of petition to authorities' is guaranteed as a fundamental constitutional right and is further reinforced by a series of protective measures.[18] For example, no one may be criminally prosecuted for the content of his/her petition to authorities if there is no prior relevant decision and explicit permission given for such prosecution by the competent authority (Article 10, para 2 of the constitution). This 'right of petition to authorities' is an essential line of communication between citizens and state authorities.

Petition to the Greek Ombudsman constitutes one aspect of the constitutional 'right of petition to authorities'. In accordance with Article 4, para 1 of Act 3094/2003, every person or legal entity or union of persons concerned may lodge a complaint with the Ombudsman, who is obliged to investigate material acts or omissions that violate rights or infringe the legal interests of the complainant. Consequently, the right of petition is not reserved for Greek citizens only, or for persons who are able to prove that they possess a legal permit to stay in the country, but it applies to all persons. It is worth noting that a significant number of complaints in languages other than Greek have been submitted to the Ombudsman. The authority is well equipped to examine complaints written in commonly used European languages: one of the basic qualifications for investigators in the authority is an excellent knowledge of at least one foreign language.

A complaint to the Ombudsman may not only be lodged by legal persons (e.g. associations, companies, etc) but also by different types of unions of persons, such as non-governmental organisations, which do not have any particular status under Greek law. The Ombudsman has already received and investigated a large number of complaints from organisations of this kind, especially from organisations concerned with the protection of human rights or the protection of some social goods.

The basic requirement for initiating an investigation is the lodging of a written complaint, signed by the complainant, which must contain the necessary personal data for corresponding personally with the complainant. In this way the Ombudsman is authorised to investigate the personal case of a citizen. It is not necessary that the complaint be submitted on an official application form: it may be written on a simple piece of paper. Furthermore, the complainant is not required to submit the petition in person. The petition can be sent to the authority via post, fax or e-mail. Thus, a simple letter, which can be sent from almost anywhere, e.g. a prison, a hospital, etc, is sufficient to trigger an investigation.

A petition to the Greek Ombudsman does not require prior appeal to the relevant public authority, or the exhaustion of all possible means of redress available to citizens. However, in practice, the authority recommends that the interested party should approach first the relevant public service, and if not satisfied by the response then an appeal can be made to the Ombudsman.

It is thus self-evident that for the Greek Ombudsman the process of starting an investigation of a case is direct, as there is no precondition of prior involvement in the process by a Member of Parliament. In addition, there is no processing fee and the services of the institution constitute a public good available equally and freely to all.

The content of the complaint

The Ombudsman may investigate a case only if its subject matter falls within his jurisdiction. In particular, the subject matter of the complaint must refer to public sector bodies that fall within the Ombudsman's jurisdiction and must in addition concern issues that the authority is permitted to examine. In the field of health, the jurisdiction of the Ombudsman extends over hospitals, outpatient health centres, and any other health-service unit which belongs to or is under the control of the state. This last category includes all health units which belong to ΕΣΥ (the National Health System) and those that belong to the (public) insurance funds or other public sector bodies. The Ombudsman has jurisdiction over all levels of the health system of the country, i.e. local outpatient health centres, provincial health centres, prefectural and university hospitals, Regional Health Systems (Πε.Σ.Υ) and the Ministry of Health.

Nevertheless, every complaint addressed to the Ombudsman must refer to a specific administrative act against which the complaint is being made. The term 'concrete act' refers to either a definite act that has been carried out or a failure to act. For example, the refusal of a hospital to issue copies of a medical file kept in its archives constitutes such an 'administrative concrete act'. Besides administrative acts or omissions the Ombudsman investigates the 'material actions' of public servants. Material actions are tangible acts, which come under the notion of administration in practical terms. This is particularly important because the full spectrum of complaints received dealing with issues of patients' rights does not refer to administrative acts but to material actions of the organs of the administration. Instances of material actions are the behaviour of administrative, nursing and medical staff, and more generally all healthcare services provided to a patient at any public-health facility. The category of material actions also includes complaints dealing with issues of malpractice. Furthermore, in this context complaints are accepted which deal with more general organisational problems of a particular health unit, or of larger sections of the health system, such as the operation of a clinic, or the emergency hospital service for a particular urban area.

Ombudsman–citizen relations

As mentioned above, the Ombudsman constitutes an independent administrative authority. This means, primarily, that the relationship between the Ombudsman and a patient who petitions is one of state–citizen. In this sense the Ombudsman is not a lawyer or a representative of the complainant in the case. Rather, the Ombudsman employs his own independent judgement and intervenes in the manner and to the extent he considers appropriate, aiming not only to resolve the particular case but also to establish the best possible procedures and practices for the future, so that repetition of similar problems may be avoided. On that basis, the expressed will or the desire of the citizen, although it is taken into consideration, does not determine the Ombudsman's actions.

Statistical recording

Two points must be clarified at this moment: first, the Ombudsman in Greece is still at a relatively early stage and it has generally become known to the public through its activities in the mainstream branches of the public administration, e.g. tax services, insurance funds etc. Thus, the public is not yet aware that every public health facility constitutes a public service, as part of the state, with everything that this entails. Second, in Greece the prevailing view of the doctor–patient relationship is one of paternalism, where the doctor, who has presumed greater knowledge, prescribes, and the patient follows his instructions. In this framework of paternalism the notion of patients' rights is a modern idea (even an aberration), and thus is viewed with indifference by a large part of the population, while at the same time it is challenged by health professionals. The patient in Greece is not always considered by the hospital staff to be a subject with rights. (Sometimes, even the patient himself/herself is not aware of this.) Therefore, the relatively small number of complaints received by the Ombudsman concerning issues of health and patients' rights must be seen within this context.

The Ombudsman began taking citizens' complaints on 1 October 1998. In the first three months of its functioning 1430 complaints were received. In the year 1999 the number of complaints rose to 7284, of which 27% dealt with issues of social welfare and health. In the years 2000 and 2001 the Ombudsman received, respectively, 10 107 and 11 282 complaints, of which approximately 30% were cases related to the work of the Department of Health and Social Welfare.

Complaints submitted to the Department of Health and Social Welfare[19]
Table 3.1 shows the number of complaints dealt with by the Ombudsman in relation to the total number submitted to the Department of Health and Social Welfare in the years 1998 to 2001.

Table 3.1 Complaints submitted to the Department of Health and Social Welfare, 1998–2001

	Total number	Complaints outside Ombudsman's mandate	Complaints resolved	Complaints resolved in favour of the complainant
1998	383	53	61	38 (62%)
1999	1991	398	1062	620 (58%)
2000	2999	906	1798	960 (53%)
2001	3322	803	2059	1098 (53%)

The vast majority of cases examined by the Department of Health and Social Welfare focused, primarily, on issues of social insurance and, secondarily, on issues of health.

Thematic distribution of cases per year

Table 3.2 shows the distribution of cases according to type in the years 1998 to 2001.

Table 3.2 Types of cases submitted to the Department of Health and Social Welfare, 1998–2001

	Social insurance	Health	Welfare	Other
1998	69%	12%	8%	11%
1999	73% (1340)	13% (242)	13% (237)	1% (8)
2000	77% (2300)	12% (365)	5% (137)	6% (197)
2001	74%	14%	5%	7%

From the total number of cases classified as belonging to the area of the Department of Health and Welfare, a large part (42% in 1999, 44% in 2000 and 42% in 2001) relates to issues of citizens' healthcare: that is, medical treatment, hospitalisation and pharmaceutical care. Similarly, an equally significant number of cases refer to issues of organisation and operation of healthcare units. Finally, in the year 2000 new thematic categories are beginning to form, such as the right to health, medical ethics, and malpractice.[20] Specifically in 2000, 13% of health and welfare cases handled dealt with the protection, or infringement, of the citizen's right to health.

Correspondingly, in 2001, of all cases handled concerning issues of health and welfare, 12% dealt with the right to health protection, 3.5% with malpractice, and 2.1% with medical ethics. Further, it is evident from the available statistical data that, in terms of gender distribution, women submitted 33.1% of the total number of cases examined in the year 2000, while men submitted the rest (66.9%). The statistics also show that over half of those who petitioned to the Ombudsman lived in Athens. From the rest only a small percentage of the complaints were lodged from abroad (notably from Germany).

The powers and limits of the Greek Ombudsman during the investigation of cases dealing with health issues

The intervention of the Ombudsman in cases which relate to the protection of patients' rights usually has a dual character: first, there is the process of investigating claims and the attempt to find a satisfactory solution for all persons concerned. Of course, sometimes it is impossible to find a solution or to correct an injustice as, for example, in the case of a patient who dies owing to a medical error. In this instance the Ombudsman limits the investigation to a simple determination of the facts and then forwards his report on the findings to the competent authorities (e.g. the public prosecutor). Sometimes, the Ombudsman requests that a formal administrative investigation takes place, aiming at the imposition of disciplinary penalties, especially when, based on the complaints made, it is found that there is evidence of liability of health officials.

Secondly, during the process of investigation, more general organisational or operational problems of any given part of the health system may become apparent. These problems cannot be solved easily. In such a case the Ombudsman takes it upon himself to recommend to the relevant service, or to the Ministry of Health and Social Welfare, new legislative, organisational or operational measures to correct existing problems or avoid them in future.

As can be seen in the 2000 Annual Report (p. 121), the Ombudsman places specific emphasis on the protection of patients' rights.

> From the investigation of cases which have been submitted to the authority it appears that the main issue relating to this category of cases [rights of patients] focuses on the behaviour of healthcare professionals towards patients and their families. Besides the well founded expectation that medical and nursing personnel should always act cordially towards patients and their families, the complainants also increasingly demand: complete, accurate and correct information be given to the patient, consent be requested for proposed therapy, free choice of physician, and a human-centred health system.

As is evident from the Ombudsman's research of relevant cases, the instances of unethical behaviour (by medical and nursing personnel) are mainly due to:

- the shortage of nursing staff
- the paternalistic attitude of the medical personnel
- the inertia of hospital officials in confronting the issues dealing with the protection of patients' rights.

Sample cases

To illustrate the process of investigation of cases which deal with matters of health, the following cases are outlined. The emphasis in these examples is on the issue of the 'right' to health protection.

A complainant requested the Ombudsman's intervention to enable his mother, who was dying of terminal cancer, to pass the last few days of her life in the state hospital.[21] The hospital had judged that there was no reason for the patient to stay in the hospital for treatment any longer since all possible medical care had already been provided. She was referred to another hospital which declined to accept her. The patient was satisfied with the treatment she had received at the first hospital and wished to stay there. The Ombudsman concluded that the patient's desire to stay in the hospital where she had received treatment was equivalent to the right for humane terminal care and the right to die with dignity. The hospital officials ultimately accepted the Ombudsman's recommendation, and allowed the patient to continue to stay in that facility. The patient died with dignity a few days later.

A complainant alleged that she had been infected with the hepatitis B virus after receiving a blood transfusion during her operation in a public hospital in Athens. The Ombudsman conducted an on-site investigation and gathered information which established that the complainant had been given a blood transfusion in the hospital. It was also found that the hospital did not take the necessary precautions to ensure that the blood used was suitable for transfusion, especially when the initial tests to which that blood had been subjected showed that it was 'suspected' of carrying the hepatitis B virus. After careful examination of the administrative and medical records, the Ombudsman reported his findings to the competent public prosecutor, as there were serious indications that the doctor in charge of the blood donation centre had committed an illegal act.[22,23] The competent court has already issued a guilty verdict.

A prisoner treated at a prison hospital protested that he did not receive any medical care, or more importantly he did not receive the correct treatment for his condition, even though prior to his imprisonment he had been diagnosed as suffering from lymphoma (cancer). The Ombudsman visited the prisoner and the administrative staff and the doctors in charge. After collecting additional information from the hospital where the complainant was last treated, the Ombudsman made a second visit to the prison hospital, this time accompanied by an expert doctor, aimed at determining the seriousness of the patient's condition and whether there was a need to transfer him to another specialist medical centre. The Ombudsman concluded that the prisoner was in need of immediate medical care that had been already delayed for a year, owing to the lack of co-operation between the prison, the hospital, the patient and his doctors. The entire system in this case seemed not to be functioning properly. Finally, after the relevant public sector bodies reached an understanding with the help of mediation by the senior investigator of the Ombudsman, the prisoner was admitted to a specialist hospital, where new tests were made on the patient and his treatment was re-assessed.[24]

The surviving daughters of a patient who died in hospital complained that they were not informed about the decline of their father's health or about the seriousness of his condition. The hospital informed them of the results of the internal investigation they had conducted, upon the complainants' request, only after the Ombudsman intervened. The Ombudsman's own investigation showed that there had been a series of shortcomings in the investigation the hospital had conducted. Most notably, the Ombudsman found that the hospital's report did not respond to the questions posed by the complainants. Their questions were about the right to be informed and give consent, the right to a dignified death, and finally the obligation of health professionals to provide unlimited medical care to a patient, aimed at the preservation of life. As a result, the Ombudsman proposed that the hospital should conduct a new investigation, with at least procedural propriety assured. This was accepted and the specific case was re-examined.[25] This case gave the Ombudsman the opportunity to propose to the Ministry of Health and Social Welfare that every hospital be required to post, in visible areas, a list of the rights of patients. In this way they could be made known not only to patients but to health professionals as well.

Analysis

Evaluation of the existing system

A determining factor in the evaluation of the work of the Ombudsman is the fact that the notion of 'patients' rights' in Greece constitutes a new category of rights which, to date, has not received wide political support, scientific elaboration or description in terms of legal precedent. Thus, it can be said that Greece has not yet developed a culture of 'patients' rights' and consequently the need for the establishment and operation of institutions and mechanisms for the protection of these rights is not fully understood. Therefore a new institution like the Ombudsman should impose its institutional presence in this field, thereby gaining not only the trust of citizens and patients, but also the approval of professionals in the field and of the health system as a whole. The development of a credible, autonomous and scientifically based authority in this field requires effort and patience. The Greek Ombudsman has so far taken steps in this direction carefully, acting with a good deal of self-restraint, as there is a danger of making a serious mistake, which could cost the institution its credibility and have detrimental consequences for its functioning in healthcare.

It is true then that the Greek Ombudsman has not developed a complete system of intervention for the protection of patients' rights. It should not be forgotten that its institutional remit stems from *ad hoc* intervention based on individual citizens' complaints. Nevertheless, the exploration of the protection of patients' rights is not only possible, but also expected. So is the formulation of an overall general institutional policy on such matters.

The questions of whether, and to what extent, the Ombudsman might have a scientific opinion on health issues have been seriously considered (provided of course that for the investigation of a case it is clear that any specific action is in accordance with the rules of medical science). Is it possible for the Greek Ombudsman to express such opinions and to formulate scientific-medical points of view? This problem, beyond its legal dimension, has a practical side as well, because within the authority's staffing structure there is currently no specific provision for doctors. One way round this problem at the moment, of course, is to use the legal power to commission an expert's report from external scientists, a power which has not yet been exercised. In the near future the Ombudsman may need to re-assess the need for permanent medical personnel who will screen cases in order to make use of this legal power. At the moment this seems to be the weak point in handling cases which involve medical malpractice.

Evaluation

Beyond parliamentary control and the daily assessment of the Ombudsman's work by the public and mass media, the Greek Ombudsman has decided that there is a need for systematic evaluation of his work. An internal and external evaluation has been taking place up to the present. The internal evaluation was carried out in summer 2000, and highlighted views on the strengths and weaknesses of the organisation and its functions and proposed ways of improvement. Subsequently, an external evaluation was sought concerning the entire work of the institution. This evaluation was conducted in October 2001, by a team of foreign experts.* Within the context of that evaluation an international workshop was organised entitled 'The Greek Ombudsman – three years of operation', but nothing has been published on these results yet. Finally, research focusing on the public's perception of the Ombudsman is currently being prepared. A third party will conduct this work, and the process of selection for a suitable researcher is underway.

Conclusion

The Ombudsman in Greece is still a fledgling organisation and so it is too soon for anyone to draw definite conclusions about its operation. In any case, the Ombudsman has already secured strong safeguards both constitutionally and legislatively, and as a result it stands on very strong ground for developing its work in the future. More importantly, it has succeeded in gaining the trust of the public and the mass media and the full support of all political powers in the country. Nevertheless, in proposing solutions which go beyond prevailing traditional standards, it faces difficulties in its relations with established administrative mechanisms. A fundamental overhaul of the entire Greek Health Services System is underway. However, the issue of patients' rights and the need for their protection have not yet gathered sufficient interest. It is precisely because these notions of rights are new social and intellectual categories in Greece that they require (with appropriate care and moderation) gradual promotion and elevation by the Greek Ombudsman.

The organisation and functions of the Greek Ombudsman do not always result in concrete outcomes and effective handling of healthcare cases. For this reason the Ombudsman's approach is still under trial until an appropriate new model for this type of case is identified. In any event, the current status of the Greek Ombudsman within the wider institutional and political structure constitutes a good platform to enable the institution to intervene more decisively in future on the debate around the protection of patients' rights.

References

1 Alivizatos N (1979) *Les institutions politiques de la Grèce à travers le crises 1922–1974*. LGDJ, Paris.
2 Dagtoglou P (1965) Die Verfassungsentwicklung in Griechenland von der Einführung der geltenden Verfassung bis zum Tode König Pauls. *JöR NF*. **14**: 381–93.

---

* Members of this experts' evaluating team were: Mr Ivan Bizjak, Minister of Justice, Republic of Slovenia, Former Human Rights Ombudsman of the Republic of Slovenia; Dr Hans Gammeltoft-Hansen, Parliamentary Ombudsman of Denmark; Dr Roy Gregory, Professor of Politics, UK, Director of the Centre for Ombudsman Studies, University of Reading; Mr Kevin Murphy, National Ombudsman of the Republic of Ireland; and Dr Linda Reif, Professor of Law, Chief Editor, *International Ombudsman Yearbook*.

3 Dagtoglou P (1983) Die griechische Verfassung von 1975. Eine Einführung. *JöR NF*. **32**: 355–93.

4 Spyropoulos Ph (1995) *Constitutional Law in Hellas*. Kluwer, The Hague and Ant N Sakkoulas, Athens.

5 Makridimitris A (1996) 'The fir tree in the sand': The Ombudsman in Greece. In: *The Control of Maladministration in Greece and in Europe*. Ant N Sakkoulas, Athens-Komotini, p. 18.

6 Makridimitris A (1995) The public administration in Greece. In: A Makridimitris (ed.) *Problems of Administrative Reform*. Ant N Sakkoulas, Athens-Komotini, SL.

7 Dagtoglou P (1993) In: KD Kerameus and PJ Kozyris (eds) *Introduction to Greek Law*. Kluwer Law International, The Hague, pp. 43–7.

8 Fitrakis E (1999) Penal law and military disciplinary power. *Iperaspisi*: 863–904.

9 Alexiadis A-D (2000) *Deontology of Health (Legislation and Jurisprudence)*. M Dimopoulos, Thessaloniki, p. 197.

10 Preamble of Law 2920/2001.

11 Ikonomou A (1996) The institution of administrative mediation and the Public Administration Investigators–Inspectors Authority. In: *'Ombudsman'. The Control of Maladministration in Greece and Europe*. Ant N Sakkoulas, Athens-Komotini.

12 The Constitution of Greece, 6 April 2001, section VI – Administration, Chapter 1, Management of Administration (article 103).

13 Inaugural speech of the first Greek Ombudsman. N Diamandouros (2000) In: *Ombudsman's Annual Report 1998*, p. 113.

14 Diamandouros N (2000) In: Citizens' Union for Intervention (ed.) *The Greek Ombudsman*, pp. 18–19.

15 Diamandouros N (2001) Introduction. In: *Ombudsman's Annual Report 2000*, pp. 6–7.

16 Fitrakis E (2000) *The investigative powers of the Greek Ombudsman (presentation)*.

17 Arsenopoulou I (2000) *The handling of cases by the Ombudsman which require scientific opinion (presentation)*.

18 Besila-Makridi (2000) *The Right of Petition to Authorities and the Ombudsman* (2e). Sakkoulas, Thessaloniki.

19 *Ombudsman's Annual Report 2001*, Athens 2002: 134.

20 *Ombudsman's Annual Report 2000*, Athens 2001: 111.

21 *Ombudsman's Annual Report 1998*, Athens 1999: 62.

22 *Ombudsman's Annual Report 1999*, Athens 2000: 114.

23 *Poinika Chronika 2002*: 944.

24 *Ombudsman's Annual Report 2000*, Athens 2001: 148.

25 *Ombudsman's Annual Report 2000*, Athens 2001: 149.

Further reading

• Alexiadis A-D (1999) *Isagogi sto dikeo tis igias (Introduction to Health Law)*. M Dimopoulos, Thessaloniki.

• Alexiadis A-D (1996) *Isagogi sto iatriko dikeo (Introduction to Medical Law)*. M Dimopoulos, Thessaloniki.

• Anapliotou-Vaseou IR (1993) *Genikes arches iatrikou dikeou (General Principles of Medical Law)*. P Sakkoula, Athens.

- Androulidaki-Dimitriadi I (1993) *Ipochreosi enimerosis tou asthenous (The Duty to Inform the Patient)*. Ant N Sakkoulas, Athens-Komotini.
- Androulidaki-Dimitriadi I (1994) *Dikeo ke igia (Law and Health)*. European Law Students' Association, Law and Health, Conference Minutes. Ant N Sakkoulas, Athens-Komotini, pp. 25ff.
- Antonopoulos M (1995) *Anexartites Diikitikes arches (Independent Administrative Authorities)*. Ant N Sakkoulas, Athens-Komotini.
- Ballas N (1995) Thesmi elenchou tis diikiseos: Ombudsman (Institutions of Control of Administration: Ombudsman). *Diikitiki Enimerosi*. **3**: 111–33.
- Charalambakis A (1993) Iatriki efthini ke deontologia (Medical Liability and Deontology). *Iperaspisi*, pp. 507–30.
- Chrisanthakis CH (1996) Ptiches prostasias tou politi stin kinotiki enomi taxi: apo ton Evropeo diamesolaviti ston Ellina Mesolaviti (Aspects of Citizen's Protection in the European Community and Greek Rule of Law: From the European Ombudsman to the Greek Ombudsman). In: *'Ombudsman'. O elenchos tis kakodiikisis stin Ellada kai stin Evropi (The Control of Maladministration in Greece and in Europe)*. Ant N Sakkoulas, Athens-Komotini, pp. 79ff.
- Enosi politon gia tin paremvasi (Citizens' Union for Intervention) (ed.) (2000) *O Synigoros tou politi: I dimokratia se vathos (The Greek Ombudsman: Democracy In Depth)*. Papazisi, Athens.
- European Parliament (Directorate-General for Research) (2001) *European Ombudsman and National Ombudsmen or Similar Bodies. Comparative Tables, 2001*. European Parliament, Strasbourg.
- Fitrakis E (2000) I akousia exetasi tou psychika astheni (Involuntary Examination of Psychiatric Patient). *Nomiko Vima*, pp. 1673–7.
- Georgiou G (1994) The responsiveness of the Greek Administration System to European Prospects. *Int Rev Admin Sci*. **60**: 131–44.
- Giannidis I (1994) *Provlimata apo tin piniki efthini ton giatron (Problems Derived from the Criminal Liability of Physicians)*. European Law Students' Association, Law and Health, Conference Minutes. Ant N Sakkoulas, Athens-Komotini, pp. 86ff.
- Kerameus KD and Kozyris PJ (eds) (1993) *Introduction to Greek Law* (2e). Kluwer Law and Taxation Publishers, Deventer, Boston, MA.
- Klamaris N (1994) *Neoteres exelixis sto thema tou varous apodixeos stin iatriki efthini (The Newest Developments on the Subject of Proof in Medical Liability)*. European Law Students' Association, Law and Health, Conference Minutes. Ant N Sakkoulas, Athens-Komotini, pp. 91ff.
- Koniaris TH and Karlovassitou-Koniari A (1999) *Medical Law in Greece*. Kluwer Law International, The Hague and Ant N Sakkoulas, Athens-Komotini.
- Kotsianos ST (1977) *I iatriki efthini (astiki-piniki) (Medical Liability. Civil and Penal)* (2e). Triantafillou, Thessaloniki.
- Koulouris N (1993) I 'anexartites diikitikes arches': ta allodapa protipa кe ta imedapa kakektipa (Independent Administrative Authorities: The Foreign Models and the Domestic Bad Copies). *Diikitiki diki*. **5**: 1140–83.
- Koutselinis A (1994) *Deontologia ke efthini kata tin askisi tis iatrikis (Deontology and Responsibility in the Exercise of Health)*. European Law Students' Association, Law and Health, Conference Minutes. Ant N Sakkoulas, Athens-Komotini, pp. 48ff.
- Makridimitris A and Michalopoulos N (eds) (2000) *Ekthesis empirognomonon gia tin dimosia diikisi (Experts' Report for the Public Administration)*. Papazisi, Athens.

- Manoledakis I (1997) Simia epafis tis iatrikis kai tis nomikis epistimis (Common Points of the Legal and Medical Science). In: *Mnimi Nikou Fotaki (Memory Nikou Fotaki)*. Ant N Sakkoulas, Athens-Komotini, pp. 123–33.
- Mavrias K (2000) *Syntagmatiko dikeo (Constitutional Law)*. Ant N Sakkoulas, Athens-Komotini.
- Michalopoulos N (2001) Methodi diikisis ke organosis ton scheseon kratous-politi (Methods of Administration and Organization of State–Citizen Relations). In: E Spiliotopoulos and A Makridimitris (eds) *I dimosia diikisi stin Ellada (Public Administration in Greece)*. Ant N Sakkoulas, Athens-Komotini, pp. 189ff.
- Mouzelis N (1978) *Modern Greece. Facets of Undevelopment*. Macmillan, London.
- Panagopoulos TH (1990) Endiknite i epanasistasi tou thesmou tou Epitropou tis diikiseos? (Recommendation for the Re-establishment of the Institution of the 'Administration Commissioner'). In: TH Panagopoulos (ed.) *Provlimatismi sto dimosio dikeo (Issues of Public Law)*. Ath Stamoulis, Piraeus, pp. 77–98.
- Papadimitropoulos D (1995) To soma elenkton dimosias diikisis, o médiateur kai i archi ton kat' epeikia liseon (équité) (The Public Administration Investigators–Inspectors Authority, the Médiateur and the Principle of Equity). *Diikitiki enimerosi.* **3**: 72–80.
- Paparigopoulou P (1994) *To dikeoma gia prostasia tis igias (The Right to Health Protection)*. European Law Students' Association, Law and Health, Conference Minutes. Ant N Sakkoulas, Athens-Komotini, pp. 76ff.
- Paraskevopoulos N and Kosmatos K (1997) *O anagastikos eglismos tou psychika astheni se psychiatrio (nomothetiki rithmisi, practiki efarmogi) (The Forcible Confinement of the Psychiatric Patient (Legal Regulation and Application))*. Ant N Sakkoulas, Athens-Komotini.
- Politis CH (1999) *Iatriko dikeo (Medical Law)*. Härtling, Athens.
- Spanou C (1994) Penelope's suitors. Administrative modernization and party competition in Greece. *West Euro Politics.* **19**(1): 97–124.
- Spanou C (1998) European integration in administrative terms. A framework for analysis and the Greek case. *J Euro Pub Policy.* **5**(3): 467–84.
- Spiliotopoulos E (2001) *Enchiridio diikitikou dikeou (Handbook of Administrative Law)* (11e). Ant N Sakkoulas, Athens-Komotini (and French version: *Droit Administratif Hellenique*, 1991).
- Spiliotopoulos E and Makridimitris Ant (eds) (2001) *I dimosia diikisi stin Ellada (Public Administration in Greece)*. Ant N Sakkoulas, Athens-Komotini (and French version: *L'administration Publique en Grèce*, 2001).
- Tachos A (2000) *Elliniko diikitiko dikeo (Greek Administrative Law)* (6e). Sakkoula, Athens-Thessaloniki.
- Theodorou M and Mitrosili M (1999) *Domi ke litourgia tou ellinikou sistimatos igias (Structure and Operation of the Greek System of Health)*. Elliniko Anikto Panepistimio (Greek Open University), Patras.
- Tsatsos D and Contiades X (2001) *The Constitution of Greece 1975/1986/2001. Comparative Approach of the Constitutional Revision*. Ant N Sakkoulas, Athens-Komotini.
- Vougioukas A (1993) *I Epagelmatiki efthini tou giatrou (Professional Liability of Physicians)*. Art of Text, Thessaloniki.

CHAPTER 4

Ombudspersons and patients' rights representatives in Hungary

Judit Sándor

Hungary, officially the Republic of Hungary or *Magyar Köztársaság*, is a mid-size country in Central Europe, with a surface area of 93 030 square kilometres (35 909 square miles), and had a total population of 10.2 million inhabitants at the beginning of the year 2001.

Introduction

The term 'Ombudsman' originates from Sweden and refers to a public office where any citizen who feels she/he has been treated wrongly or unjustly by a public authority can file a complaint. History associates the first Ombudsman-like office with Karl XII, the Swedish king who imported this institution from the Turkish Court in 1713.* Interestingly, the modern Ombudsman also has Swedish roots. It serves as a constitutional guarantee for both good administration and the respect of citizens' rights. The term Ombudsman today nevertheless often refers to various general or specialised institutions that serve for the protection of rights. They may function at various levels – parliamentary, ministry, community, hospital, etc. Without taking a position on whether these institutions should be called Ombudsman-like offices I will describe five different institutions that serve to protect the rights of patients in Hungary.

The first is the institution of the (real) Ombudsman, which is called the Parliamentary Commissioner on Citizens' Rights by Hungarian law.** It is based on public law, mainly constitutional. The second is a patients' rights model that has been introduced in the civil sphere, represented and epitomised by the

---

* Based on an interview with the Ombudsman László Majthényi by Judit Kóthy in 2001.
** None of these institutions are mentioned in legal texts as Ombudsmen; nevertheless the Parliamentary Commissioner on Citizens' Rights is regarded as an Ombudsman.

Szószóló organisation. The third alternative is the institution of the (official) patients' rights representative, introduced in the year 2000 and based on the provisions of the Health Care Act of 1997. The fourth is the patient-initiated complaint procedure within healthcare institutions. In practice, in this procedure patients often seek the help of a patients' rights representative. This possibility existed even before the 1989 political transition but since 1997 it has been explicitly mentioned in the Health Care Act. The fifth is the approach that can be used by patients when they are dissatisfied with the quality of their medical care. This was introduced in the 1997 Health Care Act. Later, in 2000, more detailed provisions were worked up but mediation still did not start to function formally until 2001.[1,2] Mediation, of course, is a complex institution, applying both civil law and healthcare law. However, in some cases it may be strongly connected to the activity of patients' rights representatives, as they may suggest patients continue their complaints within the framework of a mediation procedure.

The historical development of these institutions shows a specialisation process, which started with the Ombudsmen addressing patients' rights issues as part of their wider activities, continued with the emergence of a civil rights organisation exploring the possibility of legal regulation, and culminated in the introduction of the new network of official patients' rights representatives.

Historical background

Before describing the five major options for the enforcement of patients' rights I think it is necessary to elucidate the main elements of the post-socialist Hungarian legal–political context in which these institutions emerged.

The political and economic transition in Hungary was accompanied and accelerated by a peaceful 'civil rights revolution' in 1989. Though constitutional rights, including both negative civil liberties and positive welfare rights, were explicitly mentioned in the 1949 Hungarian constitution, in practice they were not taken seriously until 1990. The peaceful rights revolution started in 1989 when a parliamentary act* significantly extended the catalogue of rights in the Hungarian constitution.**

Though it was a relatively simple process to reach consensus on the need to reinforce political and civil rights, there was much ambiguity around and debate on the concept and future of welfare rights. The right to health, for example, was often labelled as a 'heritage of the communist past'. In fact, however, the Communist constitution guaranteed only the worker's right to health and the concept of constitutional protection of health openly substituted occupational health for health in general.[3] The widest formulation of the right to health was incorporated in Hungarian law not during the state-socialist period but during the democratisation process. Since 1989, Section 70/D of the Hungarian constitution guarantees

---

* Act No. XXXI of 1989 on Amending the Constitution (in Hungarian, 1989. évi XXXI. törvény az Alkotmány módosításáról).

** Previously, the 1949 constitution guaranteed the right to work as the basis of all constitutional rights and the new catalogue after 1989 started with the recognition of the right to life and dignity as intrinsic and inalienable rights of everyone in the territory of the Hungarian Republic.

that everyone who lives in the territory of the Hungarian Republic has a right to the highest possible level of physical and mental health. Despite the honest intent to place general health among the highest priorities of the new democratic state, both in practice and in constitutional theory, there is an uncertainty as to the extent to which this provision can be taken seriously.

In addition to the reinforcement of constitutional rights, several new institutions were introduced in the Hungarian legal system in order to guarantee respect for these rights. The most important of them was the establishment of the Hungarian Constitutional Court in 1989.[4] It provided the opportunity for citizens to challenge the constitutionality of any legal norms and judicial decisions that were based on unconstitutional legal norms. In comparison to other legal systems, Hungarian judicial review includes both pre-norm and retrospective abstract norm control. It is also accompanied by various special systems, such as the constitutional complaint (*alkotmányjogi panasz*) and the recognition of an unconstitutional situation by the failure to adopt a law (*mulasztásban megnyilvánuló alkotmányellenesség*).[5] Looking at this wide scope of jurisdiction it is no wonder that citizens, rights activists, lawyers and politicians frequently used the opportunity to file a petition to the Constitutional Court. The active role of the Constitutional Court contributed to a large extent to the shaping of the new legal regime that emerged after 1989.

Parliamentary Commissioner on Citizens' Rights (Ombudsman)

Among the Central and Eastern European countries only Poland had an Ombudsman before the political and economic transition.* Soon after the political-economic transition a very effective and popular institution among citizens was established, the Office of the Parliamentary Commissioner on Citizens' Rights. The status and competence of the Parliamentary Commissioners were established in 1993 with a parliamentary act.

There are four Parliamentary Commissioners in Hungary: a Parliamentary Commissioner for Citizens' Rights, the General Deputy and the Parliamentary Commissioners for the Rights of National and Ethnic Minorities.** This means that five years before the Health Care Act came into force the Office of the Parliamentary Commissioners on Citizens' Rights had already been created by the constitution. Though in law the 'Parliamentary Commissioner for Citizens' Rights' is mentioned, the term 'Ombudsman' is more frequently used both in the media and in public debates on this institution. The Ombudsmen are elected by Parliament, thus it follows that they are responsible only to Parliament. Apart from responding to and investigating particular complaints by citizens, each Ombudsman can conduct systematic surveys and investigations *ex officio*. The Hungarian Ombudsman system was inspired by the Finnish model, though in Hungary the Ombudsman monitors the courts.

---

* Ewa Letowska was the first Ombudsperson between 1988 and 1992.
** At the moment there is a bill in front of Parliament that would create a new Ombudsman, Ombudsman for the Future Generations. The parliamentary debate is expected in 2003.

Since 1993 Hungarian citizens have been able to turn to the Parliamentary Commissioner for Citizens' Rights for issues involving a violation of constitutional rights, whereas the institution of patients' rights advocacy established by the 1997 Health Law has been in operation for only a year.

Since 1995 a Parliamentary Commissioner's Office has been functioning in various fields of human rights. The General Commissioner has already played a very important role in the promotion of human rights by writing a report and recommendation on the situation in mental asylums in which area the commissioner diagnosed an extensive violation of human rights.

Though there is no specialised Ombudsman in the field of healthcare, the General Commissioner and the Deputy have conducted numerous investigations in relation to healthcare complaints. Depending on the contested right, theoretically any of the Ombudsmen can address patients' rights issues. If, for example, the complaint is related to the access of the Roma ethnic group to healthcare, both the Ombudsman for Minority Rights and the General Ombudsman (or Deputy) may have competence to deal with the case. If confidentiality of medical data is in question, the Commissioner for Data Protection is likely to be most appropriate. In some cases more than one Ombudsman can be involved in the process of dealing with one complaint. The main reason for the wide public recognition of the Ombudsmen is that, contrary to lengthy and costly court procedures, the investigation conducted by the Ombudsman is relatively short and free of charge. Since the Ombudsmen cannot sanction or penalise the parties, this mechanism is capable of addressing not only concrete cases of rights violations but also more general controversial practices.* In addition to the Parliamentary Commissioners there is one special Ombudsman at the level of the Ministry for Education dealing with rights of education.[6]

The Parliamentary Commissioner can deal well with problems of bad management or insufficient financing of healthcare services. For instance when emergency care is not properly organised or simply not available in some part of the country the Ombudsman may recommend a solution for numerous different healthcare institutions, including the emergency services. In an investigation conducted in Heves County, numerous violations and controversies were discovered in respect of the availability of emergency services. Since most of the issues revealed have been connected to financial problems the Ombudsman has notified the Minister for Health and the head of emergency services to re-examine the system of allocating emergency services.

The following case – which provoked a good deal of public attention – illustrates the work of the Ombudsman.

The Parliamentary Commissioner for Human Rights (Ombudsman) initiated an investigation in a case reported by several local and national newspapers.[7] In a psychiatric asylum in the small city of Törökszentmiklós (East-Central Hungary), three successive cases of fire disrupted the lives of the patients in December 2000. On the first occasion, one of the patients, Lajos Sz, who had been put in a padlocked cage,** died of smoke inhalation and burns.

Upon investigation, the Ombudsman stated that several constitutional rights were violated at the psychiatric asylum: the right to life, the right to freedom and

---

* In Hungarian *visszásság*.
** Bed from where the patient cannot move unless nursing staff open the lock.

personal security, the right to live at the highest possible level of bodily and mental health, and the right not to be subjected to torture. First of all, the use of padlocked cages is against the law, and it was especially unnecessary to restrain the patient not only by the locked bed, but also by 'chemical means of restraint', that is, sedatives. Second, the asylum directly contributed to the death of the patient. As in his room there were three padlocked cages, one of them in the middle of the room, it was impossible for the patient to escape, even in the fortuitous case of getting out of the bed after the cage burnt down. Third, the continuous supervision of patients was not sufficiently resourced at the asylum. All three cases of fire occurred in the same building, where the nurses reside on a different floor from where the fires erupted. Without any warning system such as bells, it was impossible to start the rescue operation in time.

The asylum personnel charged one of the patients with starting the fires. This was not proven, however. Moreover, because of her aggressiveness, this patient was locked in a room in solitary confinement, which violates constitutional rights, such as the right to freedom and personal security and the right not to be subjected to torture or degrading action.

It is noteworthy that during the first six years of operation of the Parliamentary Commissioner on Citizens' Rights, complaints related to controversies in the right to health and the right to a healthy environment constituted around 12 % of all cases.[8]

The need to establish special rights monitoring procedures within the healthcare system, however, was independent from this already well-functioning national office. Hospitals can be regarded as very special semi-closed institutions in which rights monitoring is often difficult. Medical documentation is not necessarily a reliable source for retrospective evaluation of medical activity.

The office of the Parliamentary Commissioner did not lose its popularity after the introduction of the institution of the patients' rights representative. The Ombudsman examines over 1000 cases annually, including different types of violation of constitutional rights. In the year 2000 the number of complaints related to healthcare rights and the rights of patients increased. This, however, may not be a reflection of the inefficacy of hospital-based patients' rights advocacy but, on the contrary, may rather indicate the success of raising rights consciousness in the field of healthcare.

Though the office of the Parliamentary Commissioner on Citizens' Rights has a good reputation and it is also very popular among citizens, it is not capable of dealing with the problems of hospitalised patients. The number of complaints that reach the office of the Parliamentary Commissioner on Citizens' Rights indicates that introducing a new model has become necessary in which hospital-based rights monitoring becomes an important element of the General Commissioner's work. In the first phase of implementing patients' rights it is especially important to provide authentic and independent help for the patients and hospitals, and also to enforce the rights that would otherwise remain empty words in the law.

Health law and the development of medical law in Hungary

Before describing the Ombudsman-like institutions specific to the healthcare sector I would like to refer to some basic elements of health law in Hungary. Regulations affecting health law have a long history in Hungary. For a time they existed as part of administrative law, although these early regulations and their related literature were only the first shoots of health law in as much as they were thematically separated from other aspects of administrative law.

Patients' rights were incorporated into the Hungarian legal system unexpectedly. The legislative process without any articulated legislative policy grew out of a paternalistic healthcare system in 1996. The Hungarian Ministry for Welfare initiated a comprehensive health law reform and by the end of 1997 the Hungarian Parliament had adopted the Health Care Act. This legal reform was implicitly based on two principles. One was to stress the new, autonomy based doctor–patient relationship. The second aim was to cover the areas of new technologies and development of the national healthcare system. As a result of these efforts a new, comprehensive act was produced by the participation of about 150 experts. In December 1997 the Hungarian Parliament adopted a new comprehensive Health Act that influenced the entire sphere of medical law. The new Health Care Act promoted the principle of patients' autonomy and provided a catalogue of enforceable rights for patients, in sharp contrast to the previous legislative model that imposed vague and often unenforceable duties on healthcare professionals. As a result of this comprehensive legal reform in 1997, for first time in the history of the Hungarian legislation a chapter in the new Health Act was dedicated to patients' rights.

A new catalogue of patients' rights

The Hungarian Health Care Act provides detailed regulation concerning some patients' rights. However, many aspects of the doctor–patient relationship still remain impressionistic. Here I describe only those rights that are listed expressly in the Act:

• the right to healthcare
• the right to respect of human dignity in healthcare
• the right to have regular and flexible access to relatives during the course of treatment
• the right to leave the healthcare institutions
• the right to be informed
• the right to self-determination
• the right to refuse medical treatment
• the right to see medical documentation
• the right to medical secrecy and right to privacy protection
• the right to enforce patients' rights
• the right to complain and patients' rights advocate.

Apart from these enumerated rights, which are mentioned explicitly as specific titles within the Health Care Act, numerous other rights can be found in the Health Care Act. The patients' rights representatives also deal with those rights. For instance the right to choose a medical doctor is mentioned in Article 8(1) of the Act, and access to religious services can be found in Article 11(6) of the Health Care Act.

Patients' rights representative*

The inclusion of patients' rights in the Hungarian Health Care Act was a difficult process. Since in everyday medical practice these rights were still alien to healthcare professionals, the drafter of the Health Act included a special additional provision, for the patients' rights representative,** with the hope that this new institution would help the enforcement of rights within hospitals.

Though the system of hospital-based patients' rights representatives has been tested before by a civil rights organisation,*** still at the time of the parliamentary debate on patients' rights the general attitude was hostile towards this new provision. Therefore it seemed sensible to postpone the time when the article on the patients' rights representatives would ultimately come into force.

Role of the patients' right representative in the Health Care Act[9]

According to the Hungarian Health Care Act, the primary function of the patients' rights advocate is to defend the rights of patients; to help them be informed about their rights; and to help them to enforce their rights within hospitals and other healthcare institutions. The tasks of the patients' rights representative include specifically the following:

- patients' rights: helping the patient to gain access to medical documentation, to formulate questions and comments relating to that
- helping to formulate the patient's complaint, and to initiate the investigation of the complaint.

On the back of a written authorisation from the patient, the patients' rights representative submits the complaint to the director of the healthcare provider institution, or to the owner of the health institution. In cases relating to medical treatment the patients' rights representative may initiate an administrative procedure and can represent the patient throughout the procedure. A further task of the patients' rights representative is to inform healthcare staff regularly about the laws on the rights of patients. Many of the patients' rights representatives have said that this service was often used by the health institutions. If this function is not exercised properly some conflicts of interest can arise, but in the first stage of rights enforcement healthcare professionals may need a good deal of help with the interpretation of new healthcare laws. The patients' rights representative can only proceed with individual cases within the framework of an authorisation received from the patient.

The representative has the obligation to call the attention of the healthcare provider's director or of the supplier of the healthcare provider to unlawful practices and other omissions connected with the functioning of the healthcare provider

---

* The general rules are included in Articles 30–33 of the Health Care Act.
** The Hungarian legal expression of 'betegjogi képviselő' can be translated also as patients' rights advocate, though I think the term 'képviselö' refers more to representative.
*** That was a model introduced by the Szószóló Foundation for the Patients' Rights.

institution across all their activities, and make suggestions for their rectification. If this is unsuccessful the patients' rights advocate has the right to take the complaint to the competent organisation or person.

The patients' rights representative gives special consideration to the protection of the rights of patients who are vulnerable because of their age, physical or mental disability, health condition or social status.

The patients' rights representative – without jeopardising the provision of healthcare services – has the power to enter the territory where the healthcare provider operates, to have access to relevant documentation, and to pose questions to healthcare staff. He or she has the obligation to maintain confidentiality relating to the patient, and to process the patient's personal data in accordance with relevant laws.

The patients' rights representative functions within the institutional framework of the capital's public health authority. He or she cannot have an employment contract with the healthcare provider which provides healthcare services for the patients they represent.

Enforcement of patients' rights

In the 1997 Health Care Act the patient's right to petition and complain to the healthcare provider was explicitly mentioned. Moreover a patient can submit a petition to the supervisory body of the healthcare institution. The healthcare provider and/or the supervisory body have to investigate the complaint and send a written report on it within 10 days. This procedure can be used independently of or in conjunction with the patients' rights representative. Since patients' rights representatives do not act in particular cases on their own capacity but always based on the authority of the patient, it might be that the patient chooses to proceed with his/her own complaint alone. It can also be that the patient seeks the assistance of the patients' rights representative at a later stage.

Since 1997 in Hungary, the law has stipulated the right for individuals to have knowledge of their options in relation to the protection and development of their health, and for making informed decisions on questions relating to their health. According to the Health Care Act, everybody has the right to information about the nature and accessibility of the services offered by healthcare providers, the rules for access, the rights of patients and the enforceability of those rights.

Investigation of patients' complaints

The patient has the right to make complaints about the provision of healthcare services to the healthcare provider and also the supplier of the healthcare provider. In both cases the complaint should be treated as part of a legal procedure within the administrative law. In practice most patients first submit their complaint to the director of the hospital; nevertheless someone may choose to direct the petition immediately to the supplier (e.g. the local government authority).

The healthcare provider, or the supplier of the healthcare provider, has the obligation to investigate the complaint and inform the patient in a written form within ten days of the results of the investigation. Exercising their right to complain has nothing to do with the right of patients to have their complaint investigated – as provided for in other laws – by other organisations. The provider has the obligation to inform the patient of this option. Complaints have to be registered and the documents relating to the complaint and to its investigation have to be stored for five years.

The 'Szószóló' model

Before the official system of patients' rights representatives was even designed, a civil rights group called the Szószóló (Spokesman) Foundation for the Rights of the Patient initiated a pilot study for testing the possibility of patients' rights representation.* This patients' rights organisation started to train volunteers even before the Health Care Act came into force. The Ombudspersons of the Szószóló Foundation** began their work in trying circumstances. The institution was practically unknown at the time in Hungary. The President of the Medical Chamber, who later became Minister for Health, and many other prominent medical chiefs openly opposed the initiative to include this new monitoring function in the health-care system. Their main fear was the loss of medical control over the doctor–patient relationship that until then had not been transparent to the general public.

In the evaluation of the trial period one criticism aired was that the Ombudsmen often could only address insignificant issues, and that the establishment of a positive doctor–patient relationship did not flow from the work of a patients' advocate. Lacking support, patients' advocates were literally left alone in hospitals.

Considering the fact that the new Health Care Act and its accompanying decrees introduce a number of new institutions and practices, certain problems of interpretation may arise in the application of the law. Therefore patients' rights representatives can play a significant role in the development of a uniform practice for interpretation in the future. They can also provide hospitals with real assistance in understanding the new legal institutions.

The Act CLIV of 1997 on Health Care does not provide an exhaustive statement, but does mention two main categories of activity. Patients' advocates are to assist patients in gaining access to their health documentation and in commenting on, or asking questions about, this documentation. They are also to assist in the formulation of patients' complaints, and may call for an investigation of these.

It is especially important that, in the unique conditions of health provision, a procedure be available within the institution in which an unbiased individual also takes part to assist in clearing up a dispute or conflict between parties. Conflicts often arise from ethical or work rights related issues, or from the vagueness of instructions given in healthcare provision. Often misunderstandings may occur as a result of miscommunication between the doctor and nurse or between the doctor and the patient. One characteristic of health provision is that it is accompanied by a great deal of risk. Failure can lead to death, permanent injury, or long-term and painful rehabilitation. The harm done by medical error also explains

---

* The author of the present chapter was one of the designers of this patients' rights advocacy model.
** The Szószóló Foundation has been in operation since 1994.

why those working in the field take criticism as an affront to their prestige, and react with a great deal of passion and fear.

Significant variations in the power and prestige of individual players in the healthcare hierarchy led to characteristically unequal competition within the field. Although relatively effective democratisation occurred at a great pace in most spheres in Hungary, healthcare has been largely unaffected by this process. In the majority of healthcare institutions, access to patients determines access to professional advancement as well as to cash tips, and who gets access to patients is generally determined by the physician directing the ward. This is why the spirit of the Hungarian health law is close to so-called rights based advocacy. At the beginning it was difficult to separate advocacy and social work, for patients' advocates are often also faced with explicitly social problems.

Patients' rights advocates should primarily help patients understand their rights, assist in the smooth practical implementation of the new legal healthcare regulations, and help resolve conflicts in interpretation that may arise between patients and healthcare workers. The experimental model provided by the Szószóló Foundation showed that it is especially important to resolve as many problems as possible between patients and caregivers within the healthcare institution.

Szószóló's cases of patients' complaints*

Table 4.1 shows the person who originated the complaint in cases investigated by the Szószóló Foundation.

Table 4.1 The person who made the complaint in cases investigated by the Szószóló Foundation*

The patient	258
The patient's relative	81
Healthcare worker	42
Doctor	27
Friend or acquaintance, anyone outside the doctor–patient relationship	24
The patients' rights representative (documentation is incomplete)	30
Manager of the healthcare institution	3
Caretaker or nurse of the patient	3

In most cases when the patients' rights representative initiated an investigation it was the patients themselves who complained. In some cases, especially in those where a patient was not fully competent, relatives asked the help of the patients' rights representative. Healthcare staff and doctors for the most part requested information about the law and its interpretation. The majority of patients complained of the lack

---

* These data are based on reports written by the patients' rights representatives of the Szószóló Foundation. In some cases the file on one anonymous patient's complaint included several other complaints, therefore the number of cases do not correspond with the stated anomalies. For instance a patient complained about the violation of more than one provision contained in the Health Act and in addition to them also was dissatisfied with the hospital food.

of channels of direct communication with the management of the healthcare institution, or with those developing healthcare policy. This was regarded as of serious concern.

Table 4.2 shows the type of complaints examined in cases investigated by the Szószóló Foundation.

Table 4.2 Types of patients' complaints in cases investigated by the Szószóló Foundation during the pilot project

Discriminatory practice in the health service	5
Ethical conflict	14
Problems with meals	19
Refusal of treatment	12
Living will cases	2
Poor communication between the doctor and the patient, withholding of information	57
Shortage of materials and technical equipment	46
Hygiene problems	10
Problems with access to relatives	11
Unsafe or careless placement or transportation	16
Inadequate healthcare provision	62
Inadequate medical treatment	63
Organisational problems	40
Problems with medical documentation: refusal to release or delay in releasing	27
Breaching the right to medical secrecy	16
Breaching the right to privacy	17
Problems with the right to leave the healthcare institution	26
Issues of respect and dignity	9
Cases of rudeness	2
Other cases	
Complaint unfounded	5
Issue beyond the competence of the patients' rights representative	4
Deception, theft, 'gratitude' payments	7
Status of valuables left in the healthcare institution	2
Cases of placing under guardianship	14
Cases concerning issues of social provision, falling within the competence of social workers	16
Damages claims	18
Cases concerning the free choice of doctor	7
Cases concerning disability pensions	11
Cases of seeking assistance	12
Cases of hepatitis C infections	7
Cases concerning the voting rights of patients	2
Cases involving a struggle between the local municipality and the hospital	1
Cases of asking for assistance in formulating petitions	1
Cases of asking for assistance in judicial proceedings	2
Cases of asking for information on various issues, such as labour law, social security, degree of disability, claims for damages	49

In the course of designing the Szószóló model it was predicted that numerous sophisticated and difficult legal problems would be revealed. In the pilot study, however, the majority of patients complained about the lack of adequate communication, access to treatment and the quality of treatment. Though patients' rights advocacy was practically an unknown institution, patients still had a good idea of how to put certain issues to the patients' rights representatives. Interestingly enough patients who are minors have shown themselves able to use the services of the patients' rights representative very effectively.

Table 4.3 groups the complaints according to specific patients' rights.

Table 4.3 Complaints according to specific patients' rights

Right to healthcare	222
Right to respect of human dignity	42
Right to maintaining contact with relatives	17
Right to leave the healthcare institution	23
Right to be informed	61
Right to self-determination	37
Right to refuse medical treatment	16
Right to access medical documentation	27
Right to medical secrecy	16
Right to privacy	17

Patients' rights representatives need especially to be able to develop, maintain and manage interaction and communication, and to develop and maintain rules of interaction (e.g., no one should dominate a meeting, and those in conflict should be able to express their views freely). Advocates often need to be able to search for inventive solutions as well. Healthcare advocates often meet with problems that are entirely new, and for which no solution has been developed. To be able to work effectively healthcare workers must know the legal background of the case and have to be acquainted with and understand each suggested solution, must be able to analyse what is common among these, and see how individual suggestions may fit together. In order to do so, they need creativity and imagination.

Patients' rights advocates must assist in finding a solution, and in the interest of reaching a solution, they must try to bring the disputing parties to give up or change attitudes that prevent the achievement of the solution. They must, as much as they can, assure that the solution reached is a personal one, and so must take into consideration the position and personalities of the parties involved. Table 4.4 shows the measures taken by patients' rights representatives in order to try to achieve the aims outlined above in the Szószóló pilot study.

It is clear from the reports of the patients' rights representatives that they often had to re-establish contact between the patient and the doctor since miscommunication was often an important element of the complaints.

The following cases from the Szószóló Foundation's experimental model illustrate the sort of complaints dealt with:

> A patients' rights advocate in Pécs was able to successfully change hospital practice when children in the inpatient ward complained that

Table 4.4 Measures taken by the patients' rights representatives in the Szószóló pilot study

Supportive listening to the patient's complaint	16
Explanation of patients' rights	52
Negotiation with the healthcare professionals concerned, attempt at mediation	202
Information exchange, clarification of misunderstandings	26
Positive recommendations for the managers of the healthcare institution	105
Concrete measures (such as initiating administrative procedures, writing letters)	44
Making contact with a relative	12
Contacting authorities and other institutions	33
Contacting an expert or independent professional	26
Convincing the patient, talking him or her into a line of action	13
Consultation, giving general information	37
Giving information on possible legal remedies	30
Assisting the patient in contacting the competent authority, institution or organisation	26
Negotiation with other organisations	3
Contacting a hospital for the patient	5
Recommending another doctor	1
Calling the attention of hospital management and authorities to the problem	4
Giving information on other relevant legal sources	2
Assistance in preparing the consent form	1
Assistance in data protection	1
Giving information on patients' rights to soldiers	1
Assistance in writing a complaint or petition, and in forwarding them	2
Contacting the chief financial officer of the healthcare institution	3
Sending a warning (on the possibility of initiating a disciplinary action)	1
Training, lecturing on patients' rights	5
Providing expert comments on patients' rights and the signing of the consent form	2
Participating and asking questions at the meeting of the guardian authority	1
Assistance in writing an application letter for receiving aid	1
Assistance in organising a meeting between the parties	1
Providing background information on the Ombudsman's statement	1
Initiating the distribution of medical equipment and donations	1

they were woken to be weighed every morning at 4:45. Because of this the children, who were in dire need of rest, were exhausted. In the course of the advocate's work it became clear that the children were woken at that hour because it had been the assignment of the night-nurse to weigh the children. In the ensuing conversation with the physician in charge it became clear that this practice could easily be changed, and so the physician in charge ordered that the children be weighed later.

In another case the healthcare advocate was also able to successfully intervene when a small child was unable to calm down after an unfortunate conversation with the visiting doctor. The child was suffering from polycystitis of the kidneys. During the visit the doctor asked the child if he knew of anyone else who had a similar disease in the family. The boy said that his grandfather had been killed by the same disease. The doctor victoriously announced to his accompanying colleagues 'didn't I say so?'!!

In cases such as the latter it is the duty of the Ombudsman to facilitate renewed communication between the doctor and the patient. No matter how difficult, the advocate must tell the doctor that the patient hears what is said about him even if it is not addressed to him. At such times calming words from the advocate are not enough, for the patient will be more convinced if he hears the doctor say that his disease can be treated, that the doctor only needed to know more about the family to understand the case fully, and that the patient will not meet the same fate as his grandfather.

It appears that children are more likely than adults to be treated as objects of examination, and not as sick individuals. During one visit a sleeping child was suddenly made to stand up. The child was terrified, and burst into tears, at which the doctors doing the rounds simply left the child. Such practice could be the result of years of indifference to which doctors working in the institution have become accustomed. It is the job of an impartial outsider with a feeling for rights and the law, such as a patients' rights advocate, to debate and bring change to such ethically questionable practices.

In one of the hospitals taking part in the experimental model, inpatients in the gynaecology ward complained that they were asked to sign their consent to the procedure about to be carried out after they had been laid on the operating table, their legs had been strapped down, and immediately after they had been given an anaesthetic injection. The list of patients registered for abortions was tacked to the wall in the hall of the hospital. These cases demonstrate that healthcare advocates often meet very severe violations of rights, including those that may even lead to lawsuits if not solved promptly and efficiently at the hospital. Here a kind of conflict of interest situation may occur as the patients' rights representative in the ANTSZ (within the National Public Health and Medical Officer Service*) model, employed within the healthcare system, still may often have to advise the patient to initiate a lawsuit against the hospital.

In practice, patients' rights representatives intervene in cases in which patients' rights are violated, or when they are treated unethically or without due consideration, but when nobody is interested in taking the case to court. The well-being, recovery, and satisfaction of patients is, however, greatly influenced by the ability to resolve conflicts within the hospital, and both healthcare workers and patients have benefited from a successful resolution of the dispute.

The years to come will show how rights and regulations established by healthcare law will work in practice. One difficulty lies in the fact that at a stroke changes have been effected in all spheres of healthcare, and there is a lack of the necessary common understanding of how to work with and apply several dozen new regulations and institutions. For a proper application of the law a thorough and ethical interpretation of it is needed in everyday medical practice, and in its application

---

* In Hungarian: 'Állami Népegészségügyi és Tisztiorvosi Szolgálat'.

in courts of law. We stand at the threshold of a new age, an age in which the doctor–patient relationship will rest upon human rights and co-operation. I hope that this change in spirit will also positively affect the most defenceless patients such as children, the mentally disabled, and the mentally ill.

The system of patients' rights representatives under the Health Care Act

When the law on patients' rights advocates was adopted, experts in the field of human rights and healthcare law strongly opposed the involvement of the public health authority in the advocacy model. They supported the creation of an Office for the Parliamentary Commissioner on Health Care. This function would have guaranteed an independent control of the healthcare system. Nevertheless, the fear of the patients' rights advocates among health politicians was strong enough to obstruct the location of this institution beyond the healthcare sector. In the first phase of the patients' advocacy model much tension was generated owing to misunderstanding the role of the patients' rights advocates.

After the very controversial first year of operation the ANTSZ started to recognise the importance of this quality-monitoring model. However, because of financial constraints the patients' rights advocates have to allocate their time between more healthcare institutions. In the capital 13 patients' rights advocates started work in 2000. This number is much below the level required. Some of them serve at eight different healthcare providers. In the rural areas, around 45 patients' rights advocates work altogether. In addition to them there is a Co-ordination Council for Patients' Rights that consists of seven members. Their main task is to control and to harmonise the practice of the patients' rights advocates.

The Hungarian Patients' Rights Council has seven members. The head of the council is charged with the territory of Budapest and each of the other six members co-ordinate the activity of the patients' rights representatives in two to four counties of Hungary. The total number of patients' rights representatives working within the framework of the public health authority is 52.* Their professional backgrounds differ, though it should be emphasised that on average they have high qualifications, including some with two diplomas. There is even one Olympic champion among them who has a medical diploma and who also studied law. Their professional backgrounds are:

- lawyer, solicitor, 18
- medical doctor, 5
- dentist, 1
- pharmacist, 1
- ambulance doctor, 2
- qualified nurse, 12
- social worker, 5
- sociologist, 1
- psychologist, 2
- administrative manager, 1
- pedagogue, 4.

* The data are valid as of January 2002.

Their activities cover 159 hospitals, primary care institutions, and medical centres. This means, unfortunately, that the patients' rights representatives work in more than one institution. In each one they have to indicate the regular office hours that they spend at the healthcare institutions. Their salary is very low and ranges from 16 000 HUF to 137 000 HUF per month (€60 to 500). Because some of the patients' rights representatives have to travel to different places it is difficult to compare the differences in their workload. Some of them take it as a part-time job but more and more of them consider it a full-time occupation.

Distribution of complaints by healthcare unit

The distribution of complaints by healthcare unit is shown in Table 4.5.

Table 4.5 Distribution of complaints by healthcare unit

Division	Number of cases	Percentage
General medical division	266	14
Surgical division	257	14
Obstetrics and gynaecology	111	6
Urology	38	2
Psychiatry	391	21
Primary care – GP	148	8
Dentistry	95	5
Neurology	84	4
Ophthalmology	29	1.5
Otorhinolaryngology (ENT)	29	1.5
Intensive care	40	2
Paediatric division	54	3
Traumatology	75	4
Pulmonology	32	2
Rheumatology	40	2
Other, less than 1% each	194	10
Total	1883	100

The distribution of complaints according to medical speciality shows quite a different picture to the medical malpractice petitions before the courts.[10] General medical care and interestingly enough psychiatry represent a larger proportion of the claims. The difference between malpractice suits and patients' complaints could be interpreted as evidence for the different use of the two procedures. It is important to emphasise these differences since many health professionals were afraid that patients' rights representatives would deliver medical malpractice claims into the hands of the advocates. Before the introduction of patients' rights representation only a few people believed that any complaints resulting would not lead to litigation.

Distribution of complaints according to the type of patients' rights violated

Table 4.6 shows the distribution of complaints according to the type of right violated. Many complaints included the violation of more than one right.

Table 4.6   Rights violated in the cases

Patients' right	Number of cases	Percentage
Right to healthcare	600	26
Right to respect for human dignity	535	23
Right to be informed	420	19
Right to access medical documentation	311	14
Right to leave the healthcare institution	61	3
Right to self-determination	123	5
Right to medical secrecy	39	2
Right to refuse medical treatment	38	2
Right to maintain external contacts	38	2
Other	80	4
Total	2245	100

The majority of patients complained about access to healthcare services and the violation of human dignity. This indicates that even the very basic needs of patients are being violated and means that patients might be prevented from complaining about more sophisticated personal requirements. 26% of complaints related to access to healthcare. This figure supports the general worry that though in theory all medically necessary health services are available based on compulsory and general health insurance, in practice, however, patients perceive that they have difficulties in obtaining adequate medical care.

Distribution of complaints by administrative area

Table 4.7 shows the distribution of complaints by administrative area, including outpatient clinics and all initiated cases even if no patient rights were involved.

40% of complaints originated in Budapest. This territorial distribution of complaints may indicate different things. It may suggest a more developed rights consciousness in the capital. But – in the light of a lack of any previous assessment of patients' satisfaction – it might equally indicate that patients in the hospitals of Budapest feel less content about the attention and care provided to them.

Table 4.7 Distribution of all initiated complaints by administrative area (including outpatient services)

County	Cases initiated		Population in the 2001 census	
	Total	Percentage	Total	Percentage
Budapest	1861	40	1 775 203	18
Baranya	117	3	408 019	4
Bács-Kiskun	65	1	546 753	5
Békés	174	4	397 074	4
Borsod-Abaúj-Zemplén	353	8	745 154	7
Csongrád	128	3	433 388	4
Fejér	143	3	434 547	4
Győr-Moson-Sopron	40	1	434 956	4
Hajdú-Bihar	305	7	553 043	6
Heves	107	2	325 673	3
Jász-Nagykun-Szolnok	26	1	415 819	4
Komárom-Esztergom	83	2	316 780	3
Nógrád	50	1	220 576	2
Pest	213	5	1 080 759	11
Somogy	133	3	335 463	3
Szabolcs-Szatmár-Bereg	131	3	582 795	6
Tolna	61	1	250 062	2
Vas	265	5	268 653	3
Veszprém	252	5	374 346	4
Zala	87	2	298 056	3
Total	4594	100	10 197 119	100

Mediation

The time and costs associated with disputes about medical negligence can be greatly reduced if the disputants are able to settle out of court. One precondition for such extrajudicial settlements to be reached, however, is that the supervisory council is unbiased and professional. Mediation was enabled by law in Hungary in 1997, but the detailed rules governing mediation were only fully worked out in Act CXVI of 2000. According to this law the healthcare provider and the patient may make use of the mediation service in a legal dispute to help reach a swift and effective extrajudicial settlement. The patient, or, in case of the patient's death, his or her next-of-kin or the beneficiary of his or her will, and the provider can request the mediation procedure. The request for mediation must be submitted in the legal chambers located closest to the patient's home, or to the health provider's office.

The petition must contain the details of the patient and of the healthcare provider, the description of the nature of the injury, the consequences suffered, and the demands made.

The healthcare provider must then ensure that the method of initiating the procedure of demanding mediation is correctly carried out, and be fully acquainted with the process of mediation. The patients' rights advocate should also inform the patient about the possibility of embarking on extrajudicial mediation.

Within fifteen days of receiving the request for mediation from one party, chambers must send the request to the other party. The other party must inform the chambers within fifteen days of receiving the request of whether that party agrees to mediation. If both parties determine to enter mediation the chambers will call upon the parties to reimburse the chambers for half the standard costs of mediation each. Once the parties have paid the costs of mediation, the chambers will call upon the parties to determine the composition of the mediating council which will carry out the mediation. The parties should choose council members from the list of qualified mediators maintained by the Hungarian Legal Expert Chamber (HLEC). One member of the council so named must be a lawyer, while the others selected from the list of mediators may hold a different higher degree. If the parties are unable to agree upon the mediator, each party may name a single member of the council. The parties may also agree that an intermediary is to present their case to the council.

The HLEC can place those on its list of mediators who request inclusion, who have a lawyer's, a physician's, or other higher medical degree, or those with higher degrees in sociological or clinical psychology, who have at least eight years' professional practice, and who have completed a legally approved course in mediation.

The council meeting is scheduled with the agreement of the mediators and the chambers, within thirty days of agreement on the identity of the mediators. Non-governmental organisations may represent the patient in as much as their constitutions state that their mission is to protect patients' rights, human rights, or advocate patients' interests. The provider may be represented by a non-governmental organisation advocating providers' rights, or by his/her professional organisation. This provision of law was warmly received by patients' rights organisations.

If the parties agree, the council may request an expert opinion. Anyone may serve as an expert who has expert knowledge of the issue at hand, and whom both parties agree may so serve. The parties may also select an expert from the list of legal experts. When possible, the expert should base his or her expert opinion on the existing medical documentation, but may also personally examine the patient if necessary. The expert should transmit his or her opinion in writing within thirty days of receiving a request for it. This time period may be extended once if agreed by both parties.

The role of the courts

If nothing else works the judicial process is still open to patients. If the patients' rights representative cannot reach an acceptable solution and the patient still complains about the quality of the medical care received, usually a civil lawsuit is initiated by the patient.

The role of the courts was an important factor in the process of adopting the Health Care Act. Hungarian judicial proceedings had an enormous impact on the development of patients' rights, though even in the context of a state controlled healthcare system patients could sue hospitals for negligence based on the provisions of *delictual liability* in the Civil Code.

The number of medical negligence cases grew significantly with recognition of the right to choose doctors. Claims for higher compensation and non-pecuniary losses have also grown significantly.

Conclusions

Since its political transition Hungary has been going through a 'rights revolution'. The Constitutional Court has been established and has started to play a very active role in the promotion of human rights. Basic elements of the rule of law have been laid down. The rule of law, however, also means the existence of a structure in which all significant players, including the government, respect and uphold the accepted normative order. To proceed to create a 'rights-friendly' attitude and environment where these new rights are implemented and protected needs enormous effort in terms of education, knowledge and creating the necessary financial resources. If the gap between rights in books and rights enforced is too wide, it leads to a devaluation of rights which may become an obstacle to the protection of basic human rights. Also it would be highly undesirable for general legal norms and provisions of the Civil Code not to correspond with the new patients' rights norms.

Patients' rights legislation is a very important tool in creating a better doctor–patient relationship and higher quality medical care. However, it also requires significant financial resources, considerate and benevolent day-to-day application, fast court procedures when necessary, and access to non-judicial dispute settlement methods (Ombudsman, administrative patients' complaint procedures etc). Patients' rights have to be consistent with other legal norms such as the duties of doctors and healthcare workers, personal rights under the Civil Code and naturally with the basic rights listed in the constitution.

Of course one cannot easily compare the practice of the official patients' rights representatives with the Szószóló model. While the ANTSZ presented a lot of aggregated data on the activity they do not have a detailed analysis of particular cases and especially about the way patients' rights representatives solve different problems. Of course it is not easy to train and monitor the activity of the patients' rights representatives in the entire country. In the future some evaluation of patients' rights representatives should be introduced. (Though formal training seems to be substantial, in my opinion it is not essential that training should include for example detailed information on first aid, sex education etc.) The major factors for success are extra-curricular, such as sensibility towards rights, problem-solving qualities and empathy.

It is to be hoped that, in future, patients' rights representatives will develop their professional integrity and independence. Since the establishment of the public health model it has been repeatedly mentioned as a criticism that the system of patients' rights representatives should be independent from the public health authorities. In the future, hopefully this independence will be achieved by the creation of a National Office of the Patients' Rights Representatives.*

---

* After completing the manuscript in March 2002, a new Parliamentary Act, (No. LVIII of 2002) was adopted that amended Article 32 of the Health Care Act. Accordingly, patients' rights representatives will work in a new organisation that will be later established by law.

Acknowledgements

I would like to express my thanks here to the hospitals who were willing to be examined in the experimental model established by the Szószóló Foundation for Patients' Rights, and I would also like to thank the voluntary patients' rights advocates who, for the first time in Hungary, took on this work. I thank Richárd Álmos, Zsuzsana Csató, Tünde Csöbi, Mária Ballay, Andrea Dallos, Márta Forrai, Mrs Katalin Juhász Gombos, Judit Hegedűs, Tibor Jakab, Eszter Kismődi, Klára László, Ádám Novák, Erzsébet Rozsos, Zsuzsa Simon, and Albert Torma. Several of them are even now working as patients' rights advocates. In order to have data about the activities of the patients' rights' representatives I prepared a detailed questionnaire for them. In the assessment of these data the help of Titusz Fábián, the lawyer for the Szószóló Patients' Rights Office, was invaluable.

I would like to express my gratitude to Dr István Felmérai, the head of the Hungarian Patients' Rights Co-ordination Council, for providing me with data on the operation of patients' rights representatives in Hungary. Research was supported by the fellowship of the Centre for Policy Studies of the Central European University.

References

1   Az egészségügyi közvetítői eljárásról szóló (2000). évi CXVI. törvény.
2   4/2001 (II 20) EüM-IM együttes rendelet az egészségügyi közvetítői eljárással kapcsolatos egyes kérdésekről.
3   Section 47(1) of the 1949 Constitution: Magyar Népköztársaság védi a dolgozók egészségét ...
4   Act No. XXXII of 1989 of the Constitutional Court (in Hungarian, 1989, évi XXXII törvény az Alkotmánybíróságról).
5   Ibid., Article 48.
6   Order No. 40/1999 (X 8) of the Ministry of Education on the tasks and operational procedures of the Ministerial Commissioner on Educational Rights. (OM rendelet az Oktatási Jogok Miniszteri Biztosa Hivatalának feladatairól és működésének szabályairól.)
7   Report No. OBH 6004/2000 of the Parliamentary Commissioner for Human Rights (Ombudsman).
8   Gönczöl K and Kóthy J (2002) *Ombudsman 1995–2001*. Helikon, Budapest, p. 228.
9   Order No. 77/1999 (XII 29) of the Ministry of Health on the legal standing of the patients' rights representative and the rules of his procedures (EüM rendelet a betegjogi képviselő jogállásáról és az eljárására vonatkozó szabályokról), amended by Order No. 27/2001 (VIII 22) of the Ministry of Health.
10 Sándor J (1997) *Gyógyítás és ítélkezés*. Medicina, Budapest, p. 237.

Further reading

•   Az ombudsman szerepe és feladatai a közép – és kelet-európai országokban a rendszerváltás után. Nemzetközi konferencia, Budapest, Nov. 21–22, 1996.

Kiad. az Országgyülési Biztosok Hivatala. Bp. Szó-Kép ny. 1997. p. 111. Bibliogr. szöveg között.

- Erzsébet R (2000) *Ápolásetikai Ismeretek*. Medicina, Budapest.
- Glasa J (2000) *Ethics Committees in Central and Eastern Europe*. Charis-IMEB Fdn.
- Gyukits G (2001) Betegjogok: beteg jogok. Betegjogi képviselet a kórházban a Szószóló Alapítvány kezdeményezése tükrében. *Beszélő*. 7–8.
- Kaltenbach J (1997) Ombudsman a nemzeti és etnikai kisebbségek védelmében Magyarországon. *Ombudsman*. 94–8.
- Majtényi L (1992) *Ombudsmann. Állampolgári jogok biztosa*. K Jogi (és). Közgazd, Budapest, p. 139.
- Polt P (1997) Az ombudsman szerepe a jogalkotásban. *Ombudsman*. 53–66.
- Polt P (2000) Az ombudsman szerepe a korrupció elleni küzdelemben. *Korrupció*. 167–76.
- Sólyom L (2001) Az ombudsman 'alapjog-értelmezése' és 'normakontrollja'. In: Az odaátra nyíló ajtó. Adatvédelmi Biztos Irodája Budapest, 2001. *Fundamentum*. 14–23.
- Varga AZ (1997) Az országgyűlési biztosok eljárásának feltételei. *Jogtudományi Közlöny*. **6/97**: 257–68.

CHAPTER 5

The Ombudsman in Israel

Galya M Hildesheimer and Carmel Shalev

Introduction

In the mid-nineties the Israeli healthcare system was revolutionised by the enactment of two major laws regulating patients' rights and entitlements: the National Health Insurance Law, 1994* (hereafter 'the NHI Law') and the Patients' Rights Law, 1996** (hereafter 'the PR Law'). Both statutes provide for the establishment of Ombudsman mechanisms.

Previously, complaints against the health system were subject to the general authority of the State Comptroller acting in his capacity as Ombudsman responsible for handling complaints against public bodies, under the State Comptroller Law, 1958.*** In addition, in the Ministry of Health an administratively appointed public complaints commissioner handled complaints regarding malpractice and disciplinary offences by healthcare professionals. Otherwise, the designation of Ombudsman officers in medical institutions and healthcare organisations was entirely voluntary.

The health legislation reform

The National Health Insurance Law

Under the NHI Law, residents of Israel are entitled to receive a comprehensive package of health services primarily through membership of one of four health funds, called 'Kupot Holim'. Previously membership in a health fund was voluntary, and in the absence of legal regulation the health funds were free to determine their obligations towards their members as they deemed fit. This gave the health funds wide discretion in admitting or rejecting candidates for membership, and independently determining the scope of health services provided to members.[1]

The NHI Law granted Israeli residents the universal right to publicly funded health services based on principles of justice, equality and solidarity. The new law specified a basic basket of comprehensive health services and medications, which residents. are entitled to receive as a minimum standard of healthcare. The

---

* *Sefer HaChukim* 1994, 156.
** *Sefer HaChukim* 1996, 327.
*** *Sefer HaChukim* 1958, 92.

primary responsibility for providing the basic basket is imposed on the health funds. However, mother–child healthcare, geriatric and psychiatric services as well as rehabilitation services are within the responsibility of the Ministry of Health. Health funds may also offer their members 'supplementary health service plans', which cover services that are not included in the basic basket guaranteed under the law as a matter of right.

In addition to the right of all insured persons to an explicit basket of health services, the NHI Law also provides for a series of individual rights. It guarantees *inter alia* the rights to dignity, privacy and medical confidentiality, and prohibits discrimination in the provision of health services. It determines the right to services of reasonable quality, within reasonable time and within reasonable distance from one's place of residence. All persons legally resident in the country have the right to membership in the health fund of their choice without any restriction, and to transfer from one health fund to another. Members have a right to representation in the health fund's council.* In case of conflict, members also have the right to initiate mediation or arbitration within the health fund, or to take legal action in a court of law. And last but not least, they have the right to complain to Ombudsman officers both within the health funds and at the national level.[2]

The Patients' Rights Law

The enactment of the NHI Law was followed two years later by the enactment of the PR Law. The objective of this law is to determine the human rights of patients and protect their dignity, autonomy and privacy *vis-à-vis* care givers. The law specifies *inter alia* rights to non-discrimination, informed consent to medical treatment, access to personal medical information and confidentiality of medical information. Most rights under this law were recognised previously in case law. The enactment of the PR Law, however, granted these rights statutory recognition.

Mandatory Ombudsman officers

This wave of legislation reflects a general human rights approach to health. However, both laws recognised that merely declaring these rights could not be sufficient. In order to realise such a far-reaching reform in healthcare an emphasis must be put on their enforcement as well. Thus, the NHI Law requires the appointment of a national Ombudsman (hereafter 'the NHI Ombudsman'), as well as the designation of a person responsible for handling complaints in each health fund. Similarly, the PR Law requires the nomination of a person responsible for patients' rights in every medical institution (hereafter the 'PR representatives').

This paper reviews the various Ombudsman mechanisms in the Israeli health system at the institutional and national levels. It is based primarily on information obtained from NHI Ombudsman's reports,[3–6] State Comptroller reports,[7,8] a survey of patients' rights representatives in Israeli hospitals,[9] and meetings with PR representatives.**

---

* The health fund council is the supreme administrative body of the fund.
** The Unit for Health Rights and Ethics at the Gertner Institute, Tel Hashomer, organised two meetings of patients' representatives of hospitals in Israel (hereafter 'The Forum'). Information presented in this chapter is based on summaries of these meetings dated 1 May 2001 and 28 June 2001, and on personal interviews with Ombudsman officers.

The diverse Israeli Ombudsman systems
The NHI Ombudsman
Historical background
The NHI Law came into force on 1 January 1995. The obligation to appoint a national Ombudsman was not complied with instantly, and it took nearly two years for the NHI Ombudsman office to be established.[10] Even after the position was established, it took some time to build the capacity for implementing its statutory function effectively, and to obtain the necessary resources for doing so, in terms of professional personnel, office space, computerisation and other technical tools. Nevertheless, the Ombudsman managed to establish a system which currently plays a major role in implementing the NHI Law and in advocating health rights.

Organisational structure
The NHI Ombudsman holds a senior and high-ranking position within the Ministry of Health. She is appointed by the Minister of Health, subject to approval by both the government and the Health Council established under the NHI Law.* The appointment is for a term of five years, which may be extended for another term of five years. The Ombudsman must be a citizen of Israel, with no criminal record and no business or contractual relations of any kind with a health fund, a health service provider, or any other corporation connected to them.**

The office of the NHI Ombudsman is an independent unit within the Ministry of Health. The only reporting requirement set forth by the NHI Law is to report the results of the examination of a complaint to the director-general of the Ministry of Health. In practice, however, she has published four comprehensive reports since her appointment.*** These reports describe the Ombudsman's powers and functions, policies and modes of action, and the areas of her purview. The reports also include statistical data and analysis of the complaints, as well as their resolution.

In addition, significant parts of the reports address the Ombudsman's opinions and recommendations with regard to the impact of bureaucratic rules, administrative regulations and legislative amendments on the rights of the insured. Among other things, she has pointed out deficiencies in the availability of information on NHI rights to the public, and emphasised the need to take measures to implement the necessity for the public to know its rights.

The Ombudsman considers that her function is to maintain a proper balance between the right to health services and the need to consider limited resources.

---

* Sections 48–52 of the NHI Law require the establishment of a National Health Insurance Council composed of 46 members representing different government ministries, various health professions, workers' and employers' organisations, municipal government, private hospitals and patients' organisations. The roles of the health council include *inter alia* advising the Minister of Health with regard to various NHI issues, conducting follow-up on the implementation of the NHI Law and publicising information about NHI rights.

** Sections 43–44 of the NHI Law.

*** See reference 2. Most of the information presented in this section is based on the second NHI Ombudsman report.

Thus, she has also addressed the need to resolve humanitarian issues resulting from the fact that essential medications for rare medical conditions are not always included in the NHI basic basket.

Role and functions

Section 45 of the NHI Law provides for a right to submit to the NHI Ombudsman complaints against health funds, healthcare providers, their employees or any other person acting on their behalf, in connection with any matter related to the law. However, although the Ministry of Health is directly responsible for providing some NHI services the language of the law excludes these services from the purview of the NHI Ombudsman. As a result, complaints concerning the basket of services provided by the Ministry of Health cannot be addressed to the NHI Ombudsman. The original intention of the NHI Law was that the services provided by the Ministry of Health would be transferred in time to the responsibility of the health funds. This has not been carried out for various reasons. So long as the Ministry of Health continues to be responsible for certain NHI services, it would appear to be necessary to amend the law so that the Ombudsman may handle complaints concerning NHI rights regardless of the identity of the body responsible for the services.

On the other hand, the Ministry of Health may be subject to the review of the Ombudsman, to the extent that it is the owner of hospitals that provide services on behalf of the health funds. In other words, the Ombudsman will handle complaints concerning services provided on behalf of the health funds by hospitals owned by the Ministry of Health. The Ombudsman has pointed out that this creates tension between the Ministry of Health and her office, which is budgeted by the Ministry of Health and is also physically located within the Ministry of Health.

As regards the Ombudsman's powers, the law states that she may recommend taking appropriate measures against respondents to complaints, and she may also attend the meetings of the health council and obtain any material related to its work. Otherwise, her powers are defined by reference *mutatis mutandis* to those of the State Comptroller acting in his Ombudsman capacity.* Thus, in examining complaints the Ombudsman is not required to comply with the rules of procedure and laws of evidence that apply in judicial procedures. She may require respondents to reply within a specified time period, hear any person relevant to the complaint, and demand all relevant information and documents from any body or person. Inquiries may be discontinued if complaints are withdrawn, rectified or regarded as unjustified.

The Ombudsman must inform respondents and, if necessary, their supervisors as well, about the investigation, and grant them the right to be heard. She must inform all the concerned parties about the conclusion of the inquiry, its outcomes and findings and the reasons for her decision. In case of a justified complaint the Ombudsman is authorised to recommend rectification of any detected defect and instructions as to how this must be done. The Ombudsman must notify the Attorney General if an investigation reveals a suspected criminal or disciplinary offence.

---

* The NHI Law refers to the duties and the authorities of the State Comptroller Ombudsman specified in sections 41, 42, 43 and 45 of the State Comptroller Law, 1958.

Operations

According to the second NHI Ombudsman report, all complaints are given a serial number and are recorded in a computerised system. In addition, complaints are prioritised and the most urgent claims are handled first. All complaints are examined by staff members with legal education.

Complaints may be submitted by phone, mail or fax. A twenty-four hour automatic phone answering service has been set up. Callers may leave a message on a private voice-mail box, and can receive a preliminary answer on the status of the complaint twenty-four hours later, after dialling the number of their voice-mail box. Personal phone answering was cut to only two hours a day to enable efficient response to urgent claims.

Where possible, complaints are dealt with and settled immediately. However, usually there will be a need for more time to complete complaint examinations, especially if assistance or information is required from external bodies, such as the health funds or Ministry of Health departments.

The reports classify complaints by subject matter. For example, the category 'basket of health services' includes complaints about access to health services, medical equipment and hospitalisation. The category 'administrative handling' includes issues such as choice of healthcare providers and delays in delivery of services, as well as violations of patients' rights (e.g. in respect of breach of medical confidentiality or access to medical information). Other categories are membership of health funds, inappropriate conduct of medical staff, and supplementary health-service plans.

After investigations are completed, complaints are classified and statistical analysis is performed. Complaints are classified as 'justified', 'unjustified', 'unresolvable' (in the case of a legitimate need for a service not included in the NHI basic basket), 'no result' (in cases of insufficient information), or 'not within the Ombudsman's authority'.

The Ombudsman's reports are usually illustrated with selected complaints and their outcomes. The second NHI Ombudsman report describes, for example, a justified complaint against a health fund that required the complainant to buy equipment necessary for surgery at her own expense. In another case, which also appears in the second report, the complainant protested against the price gap of a certain medication between different health funds. The Ombudsman concluded that the higher price was legally authorised and the complaint was regarded as unjustified.

The reports contain series of statistical tables. To illustrate the Ombudsman's workload, here are some of these statistics. According to the fourth NHI Ombudsman report in 2001, 3367 written complaints were submitted concerning various NHI issues, and 909 more had remained open from previous years. Of these, 3273 were concluded in 2001 – 26% were found to be justified, 24% unjustified, 24% unresolvable, 16% were with no result and 10% were not within the Ombudsman's authority. In addition, 1833 complaints concerning membership of health funds were submitted, of which 33% were rejected. During the first years in which the NHI Law was implemented, and following the health system's adjustment to the new legal directives, membership in health funds was an issue of major focus and was subject to many disputes between health funds and members: hence, the relatively large volume of complaints regarding registration to health funds, and their separate presentation from other NHI issues in all NHI

Ombudsman reports. According to the second NHI Ombudsman report, in 1999 5353 complaints were submitted regarding this subject, half of which were rejected.

Health funds' Ombudsman officers

Historical background

Prior to the enactment of the NHI Law complaints against health funds were handled independently by each health fund according to either the provisions of its articles of association or internal administrative rules and procedures. For example, one health fund stipulated that claims were to be submitted to its director via registered mail.

Of note was a centralised Ombudsman system established in 1973 by the largest health fund, known as *'Clalit'*.* The chief Ombudsman handled complaints submitted directly to *Clalit'*s central office, and also conducted follow-up on complaints handled by its hospitals and district offices, on the basis of monthly reports. The Ombudsman was directly subordinate to the health fund's general director to whom he reported annually, and his activity was subject to the review of the health fund's comptroller. The Ombudsman's duties, powers and operational procedures were determined by the management.[11] As for subject matter, complaints concerned inappropriate conduct of healthcare providers, long delays in delivery of services, burdensome bureaucratic procedures and physical conditions in facilities (e.g., cleanliness and over-crowding). Entitlements to healthcare services seem rarely to have been an issue.**

Following the enactment of the NHI Law, the appointment of Ombudsman officers in all health funds became a legal requisite, but it took more than one and a half years after the law came into effect for the requirement to be complied with.[12] Even after the position was established, its implementation has varied from one health fund to another.

Organisational structure

Section 28 of the NHI Law requires the health fund's council to appoint a person responsible for handling members' complaints (hereafter 'the HF Ombudsman'). Most health funds designated an employee especially for this position. One health fund, however, appointed its internal comptroller as its Ombudsman officer in addition to his existing duties.[13]

HF Ombudsmen are subordinates of the health funds' management. The national NHI Ombudsman has no formal authority over them. She does, however, meet with them periodically. Lodging a complaint at the level of the health fund is not a prerequisite for complaining to the national NHI Ombudsman, and complaints can be submitted simultaneously through both channels.

---

* Complaints against the *'Clalit'* health fund and its institutions were also subject to the handling of the public complaints commissioner acting on behalf of the *'Histadrut'*, the general trade union that owned the *'Clalit'* health fund.

** This estimate is based on a selection of complaints from 1984 reviewed by the authors.

Role and function

Section 26(a) of the NHI Law requires the health funds to set out procedures in their articles of association for submitting and examining complaints. In addition, section 28 defines the role of the HF Ombudsman as 'a person responsible for examining members' complaints, who shall indicate deficiencies that have been discovered and shall make recommendations for their rectification'. It states further that the Ombudsman shall have the powers of an internal comptroller according to the Internal Control Law, 1992,* to the extent that their powers have not been specified in the health funds' articles of association. The Ombudsman officers are thus granted access to documents and information, as they deem necessary.

Operations

HF Ombudsmen are not legally required to report on their activity, and even if they do so, it appears that the health funds consider these reports to be internal documents that are not open to the public. It is assumed that the health funds regard data concerning complaints and statistics on Ombudsman operations as confidential because of concerns about competition among themselves.

Health funds indicate the ways in which a complaint may be submitted on their web-sites. For instance, one web-site states that complaints must be submitted in writing to a specified mailing address. Another web-site introduces an e-mail method for complaint submissions, by means of a complaint form that is displayed on the site.

Patients' rights representatives**

Historical background

Prior to the PR Law there was no legal or administrative requirement to nominate Ombudsman officers in medical institutions. Some institutions, however, did informally appoint a person in charge of handling complaints. In 1996, following the enactment of the PR Law, it became a legal requirement to designate a patients' representative in medical institutions.

Organisational structure

Section 25 of the PR Law requires the director of every medical institution to designate an employee 'responsible for patients' rights'. Section 1 of the PR Law defines 'medical institutions' as hospitals or clinics.

At the level of the health funds it seems as if the Ombudsman officers appointed under the NHI Law operate also as PR representatives as regards the clinics operated by the health fund. This is possible since the NHI Law does not restrict the power of HF Ombudsmen to the handling of complaints that only concern NHI issues. At the same time, it appears that hospitals owned by health funds have complied independently with the requirement of the PR Law and appointed their own PR representatives.

---

* *Sefer HaChukim* 1992, 198.
** The content of this section is based primarily on information presented by Kismodi and Hakimian (*see* refs. 7 and 8) and on summaries of meetings of the Forum (*see* ref. 9).

As for hospitals, it appears that most complied formally with the law and appointed PR representatives, but full-time appointments are not the norm. In many hospitals the PR representative holds an additional position, such as chief social worker, physician, legal adviser or public relations officer. In more than one case, hospital directors appointed themselves* as PR representatives.[14] In one hospital, the PR representative is the person responsible for insurance risk management. Clearly, many of these dualities within the institution give rise to conflicts of interest.

The PR Law does not specify any requirements in terms of professional or educational qualifications. It appears that none of the PR representatives received special training prior to their appointment.[15]

Role and function
Section 25 of the PR Law defines the functions of the PR representative as threefold:

1   to provide patients with counselling and assistance in realising their rights
2   to receive, investigate and handle patients' complaints
3   to instruct and educate the medical and administrative staff of the institution with regard to the provisions of the PR Law.

However, it appears that many PR representatives focus mainly on the handling of complaints, and disregard their statutory duties to act as patient counsellors and hospital staff educators.[16]

The PR Law sets forth a series of patients' rights including: the right to appropriate medical treatment, non-discrimination in healthcare, information regarding the identity of care givers, the right to a second medical opinion, continuity of care between medical institutions, the right to be visited during hospitalisation, dignity and privacy, emergency medical care, informed consent to medical treatment, access to personal medical information and medical confidentiality.

PR representatives also handle complaints regarding what may be termed 'consumer issues' (such as parking, food and laundry facilities), as well as inappropriate conduct of hospital staff, and problems concerning hospital fees and health insurance issues.[17]

Operations
The PR Law does not specify the ways and means for carrying out representatives' duties. Thus the operational capacity of the PR representatives depends largely on the good will of the hospital management. Many representatives claim they do not have the power they need to examine complaints. Some of them express frustration concerning their inability to do more.[18] Indeed, there appear to be vast differences between the activities of different patients' representatives. Whereas some are minimal, the work of others reflects both professional competence and sincere dedication to the promotion of patients' rights. More importantly, their ability to work effectively depends on several external factors,

---

* This practice, beside being inappropriate, seems incompatible with the language of the law. Section 25(2) of the PR Law indicates that representatives must refer complaints regarding quality of healthcare to be handled by the director of the medical institution. Hence, the position of the institution's director and that of the patients' representative are to be separate and can not be combined.

including the extent of the management's support and co-operation, the financial, human and technological resources at their disposal, and their professional training.[19]

Complaints may be submitted orally or in writing, formally or informally. Not all hospitals have clear procedures as regards methods and avenues for complaint submissions, or timetables and directives for their investigation and handling. Most PR representatives computerise the collected data and utilise it for internal needs to improve hospital services. However, complaints are not documented in all hospitals. Likewise, not all PR representatives deem informal or oral complaints as worthy of official recording.[20]

The law neither mandates reporting by PR representatives, nor requires transparency of their activities and data. Information on the subjects of complaints, their handling and the data gathered and analysed by the representatives is all considered by the hospitals to be internal documentation, and is not published in any way. Therefore, accurate data concerning the volume and nature of complaints do not exist.[21]

PR representatives employ different methods of work, aside from handling complaints. These include follow-up of complaints in discussions with staff members (especially in departments with relatively high complaint rates), unannounced inspections in hospital departments, making sure all healthcare staff wear name tags, posting notices and handing out brochures regarding patients' rights, providing a toll-free phone number by which they can be reached, handing out questionnaires to patients, or conducting focus groups to assess patients' satisfaction.

Other good practices concerning personnel education include conferences and annual workshops for doctors, nurses, administrators and other hospital staff, multi-day training sessions for new medical and nursing staff, publishing information on patients' rights in hospital journals, as well as organising seminars and lectures given by professionals.[22]

In the *Clalit* health fund, a group of hospital representatives convenes on a regular basis to share experiences, discuss common problems and exchange ideas for good practices. The group also conducted a survey of implementation of the PR Law in *Clalit* hospitals.*

According to section 25(2) of the PR Law, complaints regarding 'quality of care' are excluded from the purview of PR representatives, and must be referred to the director of the medical institution (a physician).** The law does not define the term 'quality of care', leaving it open to varying interpretations. However, the common understanding is that it means professional standards of medical care. Hence, complaints that might evolve into legal action for medical malpractice or other types of liabilities (e.g., injuries in hospital grounds), and require the involvement of lawyers and risk management personnel, are not handled by PR representatives. The position of the Israel Medical Association, however, is that 'quality of care' includes ethical issues, which are, in its opinion, an integral part of medical care. According to this view patients' representatives are empowered to deal only with

---

* This information was obtained through a personal meeting with the Ombudsman of the *Clalit* health fund and other persons responsible for this survey.

** At the time the PR Law was enacted, the Public Health Ordinance, 1945 provided that the head of a hospital must be a medically trained professional. Since then, the ordinance has been amended to allow for persons with health management professional training to assume this position.

complaints regarding procedural and administrative aspects of the PR Law, and are disqualified from dealing with ethical matters, which are to be handled solely by either the Ministry of Health or the medical association itself.[23] However, this interpretation seems to deviate from the legislative intention. The term for 'patients' representative' in the PR Law is 'person responsible for patients' rights'. Patients' rights surely include ethical issues and not only minor complaints or concerns regarding procedures or administration.

The Ministry of Health Commissioner[*]

Historical background

In 1976 the Ministry of Health established the office of the 'Public Complaints Commissioner' (hereafter 'the Ministry of Health Commissioner'). The commissioner is an administrative appointment, and the position as such is not regulated by any law, although it appears that the Public Health Ordinance, 1940[24] sets its statutory terms of reference. In the case that a complaint about a violation of patients' rights comes to the knowledge of the Minister of Health, he may appoint a governmental doctor to examine the patient's medical records, and the medical institution must provide all information necessary for investigating the case.[**]

Organisational structure

Since 1994 the Ministry of Health Commissioner has acted within the Division of Quality Assurance at the Ministry, and is technically subordinate to the head of the division.

The commissioner is a medical professional with a part-time position. The fact that he acts within the Ministry of Health, and at the same time also examines complaints against hospitals owned by the ministry, may lead to conflicting interests. The commissioner himself, however, states that his objectivity is not affected, although he will not handle complaints concerning the particular medical centre with which he is affiliated.

The NHI Ombudsman and the Ministry of Health Commissioner currently operate independently at the Ministry of Health side by side. Although they may refer complaints to each other, they do not co-operate in the actual handling of complaints. Similarly, the Ministry of Health Commissioner has no working relations with HF Ombudsman officers or PR representatives in medical institutions, and they rarely address him or refer complaints for his examination.

Role and functions

The commissioner handles complaints against the health system from any source. Most complaints regard medical malpractice and disciplinary offences by health professionals. The definition of 'disciplinary offence' in the Physicians Ordinance

---

[*] The content of this section is based primarily on information received from the commissioner himself, and a review of his work published in State Comptroller reports.

[**] According to section 29A(3) of the Public Health Ordinance, a governmental doctor examining complaints regarding violation of patients' rights on behalf of the Minister of Health is empowered to examine patients' medical records, and medical institutions are obliged to provide all information required to execute complaint inquiries.

[New Version], 1976*,25 includes any conduct unbefitting the medical profession. Hence, the commissioner considers himself to be authorised also to handle complaints concerning violations of rights guaranteed under the PR Law. In this domain the operations of the commissioner and the NHI Ombudsman overlap, as a result of overlapping legal provisions of the PR Law and the NHI Law. For example, the NHI Law determines that health services be provided with due respect for human dignity, protection of privacy and preservation of medical confidentiality. The NHI Ombudsman is therefore authorised to handle complaints concerning these issues. However, these rights are also stated in the PR Law, which was enacted two years after the enactment of the NHI Law. Due to this overlap, both Ombudsman officers would handle complaints regarding patients' rights upon receiving them. In all other domains they would transfer to each other complaints submitted to them but coming under the authority of the other Ombudsman. In addition, all lawsuits filed against health practitioners are brought to the commissioner's attention, so that he may recommend taking disciplinary action, if he deems this necessary.

Despite the terms of reference in the Public Health Ordinance, the commissioner claims that in practice he lacks authority and tools to perform his functions and to ensure the co-operation of medical institutions in investigating complaints. Although most medical institutions voluntarily respond when approached by the commissioner, his dependence on their good will is a burden on his activities and may cause delays in handling complaints.

The legal department of the Ministry of Health has for several years been working on draft legislation designed to reform disciplinary proceedings against physicians. The latest version includes provisions for the appointment of a medically qualified commissioner, who shall be empowered to investigate disciplinary offences. The definition of a 'disciplinary offence' expressly includes violations of patients' rights under the PR Law. The bill also states that the powers of the commissioner shall not detract from those of the NHI Ombudsman and the State Comptroller.**

Operations

Each complaint received at the commissioner's office is documented and computerised. Confirmation of receipt of the complaint is sent to the complainant. The respondent is asked to reply to the claim, and the relevant medical records are ordered from the medical institutions. The commissioner then presents the gathered information to an advisory team, which studies and analyses it with a view to a joint decision. Expert opinions may also be called for. Once the facts are clarified the commissioner may recommend either sending the respondent a letter of reprimand, or the appointment of a committee of inquiry to collect additional information and carry out an in-depth investigation. If the findings of the inquiry committee reveal grounds for disciplinary procedures, the case is referred to a hearing before a disciplinary tribunal, which may recommend disciplinary measures. The final decision lies with the Minister of Health.

---

* The original version of this bill, published in *Haza'ot Chok* 1998, 318, has undergone significant amendments in parliamentary committee.
** The latest version of the bill is pending its final reading in the Knesset, but the chances for its actual enactment are unclear.

The handling of a complaint may last several months and sometimes even up to two years, depending on the complexity of the case, the co-operation of the medical institution and the availability of inquiry-committee members. According to the official data recorded at the Ministry of Health Commissioner's office, during the years 1995 to 2001 the commissioner handled an average of 725 complaints annually.

The State Comptroller Ombudsman*

The Ministry of Health, the health funds and public hospitals are all subject to the review of the State Comptroller. According to section 46(e) of the NHI Law the powers of the NHI Ombudsman at the Ministry of Health do not detract from the general powers and functions of the State Comptroller as Ombudsman to handle complaints regarding the health system. Thus, the State Comptroller continues to receive and handle complaints regarding healthcare, and health rights and entitlements. Only if a case regards purely medical issues, which require medical investigation, does the State Comptroller advise the complainant to address her claim to the Ministry of Health Commissioner. The State Comptroller also handles complaints lodged against the Ombudsman officers in the health system themselves. In these cases the State Comptroller inquires if the Ombudsman officers acted reasonably, and if they exercised their powers fairly and effectively.

The number of complaints regarding the health system handled by the State Comptroller is much lower than that of the complaints handled by the NHI Ombudsman. For example, between September 2000 and December 2001 the State Comptroller Ombudsman received 191 complaints against the Ministry of Health and 128 complaints against health funds.[26]

Conclusions and recommendations

The Israeli healthcare system contains several Ombudsman mechanisms. Complaints can be submitted at the level of the medical institution where healthcare is delivered, at the level of the health funds responsible for providing NHI services, at the level of the Ministry of Health – to the NHI Ombudsman or the public complaints commissioner – or at the level of the State Comptroller. Individuals may lodge complaints through different channels simultaneously, according to their personal convenience. Thus, submitting a complaint to the health fund or medical institution Ombudsman is not a prerequisite to complaining at the level of the Ministry of Health.** Moreover, the various Ombudsman officers act independently of each other, with little, if any, co-ordination, collaboration or co-operation. This may lead to situations where different Ombudsman officers may unknowingly handle the same complaints at the same time.

---

* The content of this section is based primarily on information obtained from the person responsible for complaints against the health system in the State Comptroller office.

** Similarly, submitting a complaint to an Ombudsman is not required before taking legal action or initiating arbitration or mediation within health funds.

Whereas in the past the number of complaints lodged against the health system was relatively low, the new health legislation and the establishment of formal channels for complaint submission increased consumer awareness of health rights, and the volume of complaints grew dramatically. Hoshen and Marx claim that previously only few bothered or even dared to complain to medical institutions or to the Ministry of Health. They explain that patients feared their complaints would be held against them while they are still in need of health services. Furthermore, few patients were acquainted with complaint submission procedures, and many were skeptical as to whether complaining would do any good.[27] However, owing to the fact that Ombudsman officers operating in health funds and in medical institutions do not publish information regarding their workload, statistical data are available only with regard to the work of the Ombudsman officers of the Ministry of Health and the State Comptroller. Moreover, figures published by Ombudsman officers may overlap. Therefore, an accurate picture of the overall workload of Ombudsman officers within the Israeli health system is unavailable.

In sum, it appears that the new legislative requirements regarding the appointment of mandatory Ombudsman officers are of major importance and benefit. Yet, further research is needed in order to assess their actual contribution to the health system, and to determine how much the residents of Israel know about the Ombudsman systems and value their operations.

In the light of all the above, we can conclude with the following recommendations. Some already exist to a certain degree within the different Ombudsman systems, and if so, it is suggested that they be applied system-wide.

1 Ombudsman officers should meet regularly to exchange working methods and good practices, share their experiences and assist each other in resolving common difficulties.
2 A professional forum could also produce a standardisation of Ombudsman procedures and record-keeping. This would allow for consistency in the operation of different Ombudsman officers, and for comparison and analysis of data collected by them, and would also enhance the efficiency of the overall system.
3 Standardisation of procedures for submitting and handling complaints would also make the system more accessible and effective for complainants.
4 The public also needs information on the very existence of Ombudsman officers, and on how they can be contacted for the submission of a complaint.
5 Professional qualifications for Ombudsman officers should be defined by law to ensure basic competence.
6 Ombudsman officers would benefit much from ongoing training and continuing education programmes in the areas of health rights, communication skills, conflict resolution and administration.
7 Ombudsman officers should be employed in full-time positions, so that conflicts of interest with other duties to the employer do not exist.
8 Adequate budgets and other resources necessary to the efficient operation of an Ombudsman system should be allocated so as to guarantee administrative and professional independence.
9 Periodic reporting on Ombudsman activities and results should be mandatory. The reports should be open to public review.

References

1 State of Israel (1990) *Report of the State Commission of Inquiry into the Operation and Efficiency of the Healthcare System in Israel*. pp. 40–2.

2 Shalev C and Chinitz D (1997) In search of equity and efficiency: health care reform and managed competition in Israel. *Dalhousie Law J.* **20**: 553–82.

3 State of Israel, Ministry of Health (1998) *National Health Insurance Law Ombudsman, Annual Report 1 for the Year 1997* ('the first NHI Ombudsman report').

4 State of Israel, Ministry of Health (2000) *National Health Insurance Law Ombudsman, Report Number 2 for the Years 1998–1999* ('the second NHI Ombudsman report').

5 State of Israel, Ministry of Health (2001) *Ombudsman, Report Number 3 for the Year 2000* ('the third NHI Ombudsman report').

6 State of Israel, Ministry of Health (2002) *Ombudsman, Report Number 4 for the Year 2001* ('the fourth NHI Ombudsman report').

7 State of Israel, State Comptroller (1997) *Annual Report 47 for the Year 1996 and for Fiscal Year 1995* ('State Comptroller Report 47').

8 State of Israel, State Comptroller (1998) *Annual Report 48 for the Year 1997 and for Fiscal Year 1996* ('State Comptroller Report 48').

9 Kismodi E and Hakimian R (2001) A survey of patients' rights representatives in Israeli hospitals: 1999–2000. *Medicine and Law.* **20:** 17–36 ('Kismodi and Hakimian' or 'the Survey').

10 State Comptroller Report 48, op. cit., p. 165.

11 Health Fund of the General *Histadrut* Trade Union in Israel, the Internal Controller (1990) *Review Report: The Handling of Members' Claims and Complaints in Health Funds' Institutions.* Tel Aviv.

12 State Comptroller Report 48, op. cit., p. 164.

13 Ibid.

14 Kismodi and Hakimian, op. cit., p. 20.

15 Ibid., p. 21.

16 Ibid., p. 29.

17 Ibid., pp. 24–5.

18 Ibid., pp. 29–30.

19 Ibid., p. 30.

20 Ibid., pp. 22–4.

21 Ibid., p. 26.

22 Ibid., pp. 26–7.

23 Israel Medical Association (1996) *The Patients' Rights Law, 1996.* Ramat Gan, p. 36.

24 *Palestine Gazette.* **Suppl. 1**, (h) 116, (e) 154.

25 *Dinei Medinat Yisrael.* 594.

26 State of Israel, Ombudsman (2002) *Ombudsman Annual Report 28,* p. 87.

27 Hoshen Y and Marx A (1997) *One Minute Doctor… A Guide to Patients' Rights in Israel.* Ethics Publishing Company, Tirat HaCarmel, p. 207.

CHAPTER 6

The Norwegian Patient Ombudsman scheme

Olav Molven

Introduction

To fully understand the Norwegian Patient Ombudsman scheme, some contextual knowledge is required about the framework within which the Ombudsman works. Before describing and discussing the scheme, this section starts with a brief overview of the healthcare system, health legislation and the supervisory and compensation system in Norway.

Background and administrative framework

The healthcare system

Norway has about 4.5 million inhabitants. The country is divided into 19 counties with populations ranging from 75 000 to 500 000. The counties are further divided into municipalities with populations between 240 and 500 000. There are 435 municipalities. The capital, Oslo (pop. 500 000), regarded both as a county and a municipality, is included in these figures. The boards of both the counties and the municipalities are appointed through general elections. The national state authorities control overall policy design and the capacity and quality of healthcare through budgeting and legislation. The state also finances a national insurance scheme covering each citizen in a uniform way. All residents are entitled to the same services, and these services must legally be provided to a minimum standard. The provision of healthcare has for many years been based on a decentralised public model. Until 2001, counties were responsible for secondary (specialised) healthcare, including somatic and psychiatric hospitals, and municipalities were responsible for primary care. From 2001 this model has been modified.

Today the state assumes responsibility for delivering secondary care, this function being delegated to five regional state-owned healthcare enterprises, each with their own board. Each of the five regional enterprises covers a defined part of the country, and is relatively free to organise the provision of services as it sees fit, provided this conforms to legal requirements.

Municipalities remain responsible for primary care. This includes general practitioners, midwifery, a central emergency call-line, home nursing care, nursing homes, physiotherapy and both individual and environmental preventive healthcare. Recently, a population-based fixed list system for general practitioners was put in place. Counties are now responsible only for children's dental services, the elderly and people with disabilities.

Health legislation

Laws are enacted by Parliament. If explicitly specified in written law, the national government or a ministry is given authority to issue more detailed regulations on specified topics. In practice, while statutes lay down the legal framework, they also go a long way towards regulating more specific issues. Regulations tend to supplement statute, especially on technical matters, but as a general rule, they play a minor role in Norwegian health law.

Over the last 50 years, and especially the last 20 years, issues of healthcare and in particular questions concerning patients' rights have been under debate. As a result, the health service has been subject to increased political control. In the beginning the state's contribution to the health service was primarily financial. Since 1980 legal regulations have played a more significant role.

In principle the legislation has been organised in five areas that regulate respectively:

1 the financing of health services
2 the relevant administrative body responsible for health services, and of the minimum range of services to be provided
3 the relationship between these institutions/bodies and healthcare staff employed by them
4 the relationship between citizens/patients and these institutions
5 the relationship between patients and healthcare staff.

The year 2001 saw significant reform of health legislation. An important part of this reform was to introduce a small number of comprehensive statutes. Each statute governs major elements of the healthcare system and its operation, and collectively they cover almost all aspects of health. It is perhaps fair to say that we now have nine main health laws:

1 the Social Security Act
2 the Municipal Health Services Act
3 the Specialised Health Services Act
4 the Mental Health Care Act
5 the Health Care Personnel Act
6 the Patients' Rights Act
7 the Act on Communicable Diseases
8 the Supervision Act
9 the Act on Patient Compensation.

Patients' rights

During the 1980s and the 1990s patients' rights developed into a central concept within public debate. At the end of the 1990s this culminated in the Act on Patients' Rights. Not only are citizens given different rights as patients, but they also have the right to become a patient when specific conditions are met, including the right to publicly funded consultations and treatment.[1]

To safeguard patients' interests, legislation has increasingly been developed in accordance with the principle of rights and duties.[2] Those who have duties are mainly the municipalities, the state and the different health professions. Citizens and patients have rights corresponding to these duties. Therefore, what is described as a right in the Act on Patients' Rights is correspondingly described as a duty in acts relating to municipal health services, secondary health services and health personnel. Though some rights may be considered vague, many are very specific. The right–duty system also gives rise to the fact that patients who consider their rights have been infringed may have their cases reviewed by the County Medical Officer or in court (*see* p. 94).

The Act on Patients' Rights sets out a series of rights for patients.[3–5] Basically, patients have the right to consultation and treatment, together with a free choice of physician and of hospital. It is expressed as a duty both in the Health Care Personnel Act, the Municipal Health Services Act and the Specialised Health Services Act that services must be of a minimum standard, i.e. they must be of reasonable quality. Furthermore, patients do, for example, have the right to participate in treatment decision-making, the right to informed consent to medical treatment, the right to access to medical records, the right to have a copy of their records and the right to medical confidentiality. Importantly for the purposes of this chapter, patients also have the right to complain when they think their rights have been violated.

Citizens' rights to hospital treatment will from 2004 be considerably strengthened.* Hospitals will no longer be able to use 'lack of capacity' as a reason for not giving health services to patients that otherwise fulfil the criteria set by the law for having the right to treatment. The state-owned healthcare enterprises will from that time have a duty to provide specialised health services by sending such patients abroad to get treatment, and the enterprises themselves will have to pay for it.

The rule of law

Certain measures have been designed specifically to ensure that these laws are put into practice.

1   It is a legal obligation for those providing health services to establish an internal control system, i.e. to establish systematic measures to ensure and document that activities are performed in accordance with requirements laid down by legislation or regulations. These systematic measures must be specified in administrative procedures.
2   A supervisory authority – an independent state board, The Norwegian Board of Health, including 19 County Medical Officers – is responsible for overseeing

---

* Proposition No. 63 (2002–03) to the Odelsting (Parliament). About the Act on Patients' Rights. (Only in Norwegian.)

health services and health workers. The board determines whether healthcare providers have an appropriate internal control system, and whether services comply with law and regulation.

3 According to the Act on Patients' Rights § 7-1 patients who are not satisfied and think their rights have not been met have the right to ask those with the corresponding duties of service to revisit their decisions. They have a duty to give an answer.

4 Patients who believe their rights have been violated also have the right to complain to the County Medical Officer. This officer has the power to reverse a decision made by the health service or by health personnel, and may also institute disciplinary proceedings.

5 Patients who have suffered personal injury may present their case to the patient compensation scheme.

6 To safeguard patients who need assistance in securing their rights, there are both the Parliamentary Ombudsman and 19 regional Patient Ombudsmen.

The supervisory authority/the county medical officers

The supervisory authority has its legal basis in the Supervision Act. The Norwegian Board of Health is the central element of the supervisory authority. This is a professional agency under the Ministry of Health. For technical matters, this board is an independent body, and the ministry cannot instruct or overrule the board in individual cases. There are approximately 80 employees; about half of them are health personnel, and the rest are lawyers and others. The County Medical Officers, each staffed with between 12 and 20 employees, represent the local supervising authority. These officers perform the practical supervision of the health professionals.[6]

According to § 7-2 of the Act on Patients' Rights, patients are entitled to have virtually all decisions made by the health service or health personnel, concerning rights to health services, information, consent and documentation, reviewed by the County Medical Officer. § 7-2 states:

> If the healthcare provider rejects the request, or if it is of the opinion that its duty has already been carried out, a complaint may be submitted to the County Medical Officer. The complaint shall be sent to the County Medical Officer.

The County Medical Officer has the power and the duty to reverse any decision that is not in accordance with the law. Decisions made by the supervisory authority may be brought to the court.

Patients also have a right to have cases tried even where there is no specific decision or act to reverse. In such cases, the County Medical Officer must always consider the patient's views, and determine whether the law or regulations have been violated, i.e. whether treatment has held to a minimum standard. As stated in § 55:

> A person, who is of the opinion that provisions relating to duties stipulated in or pursuant to this Act have been breached in his disfavour,

may request an assessment of the matter from the supervising authority. The patient may act through a representative. The request is to be sent to the County Medical Officer.

The County Medical Officer shall consider the views put forward in the request, and may also address other matters than those put forward in the request.

At the end of the case, the County Medical Officers must provide a decision where it is stated whether the law has been broken or not, and they should if requested give guidance.

The Norwegian Board of Health is responsible for co-ordinating the County Medical Officers and their uniform application of the law throughout the country. In serious cases the County Medical Officers are obliged to report to the National Board of Health. If they are of the opinion that health professionals have negligently contravened their duty in the Act on Health Personnel, and the breach of this duty is liable to endanger the safety of health services or impose a considerable burden on patients, they have such a duty. The National Board of Health has the power to give the relevant health professional a warning or, in very serious cases, to withdraw their licence to practise.[7]

The patient compensation scheme

This scheme has its legal basis in the Act on Patient Compensation.[8] It covers all patients receiving any form of healthcare from any private or public health service. This includes, for example, patients receiving healthcare from doctors, nurses, midwives, dentists, physiotherapists, pharmacies, orthopaedic practitioners and in ambulances. The principal element of the law is to determine whether or not a hospital or medical professional has failed in its duty when a patient has suffered injury, even if no one is at fault. There are also circumstances set out in the law which establish liability even where there has been no failure; in specific situations there is strict liability. This means we should perhaps characterise the scheme as an arrangement somewhere between a no-fault and a malpractice system.

To obtain compensation there must also be a proven causal connection between the incorrect treatment and/or diagnosis and the alleged injury. In some situations it is not necessary to *prove* a causal connection between the treatment and the damage. For example it is stated in the Act on Patient Compensation § 3:

> If the cause of damage to a patient's health cannot be established and the damage is in all probability attributable to an external influence during the treatment of the patient, it shall be assumed that the damage is caused by fault or failure in the provision of health services.

According to the law both physical and psychological damage are included.

The patient compensation scheme is a neutral body comprising approximately 40 claims handlers and about 10 medical doctors in the role of medical advisers. In addition it obtains expert assessment from independent professionals in nearly half of all cases. Patients who are not satisfied with the decision may appeal to a special board, and may ultimately have the case tried in court.

The Civil Ombudsman

Norway was one of the first countries to set up an Ombudsman scheme. The Parliamentary Ombudsman for Public Administration (hereafter named Civil Ombudsman) was in place as early as 1962. The reason for this was simple: public administration had already become a huge body within the framework of the welfare state. Most citizens had to interact with this public administration, and felt powerless as individuals in the face of such a large organisation. An independent body was needed to carry out investigations without having to resort to protracted court battles. Consequently, Parliament elects a Civil Ombudsman, who is accountable to Parliament.

The task of the Civil Ombudsman is to ensure that injustice is not committed against any individual by the public administration, by civil servants or by any other person working within the service of the public administration.

The intervention of the Ombudsman follows a complaint or can be by his own initiative. Any person who believes he or she has been subject to injustice by public administration has the right to bring a complaint to the Ombudsman. Likewise any person who has been deprived of his or her personal freedom is entitled to complain to the Ombudsman. At the end of the case-handling the Ombudsman must provide a decision in which he gives his opinion on the issues relating to the case. In practice, when the Civil Ombudsman expresses a point of view, the public authority responds to this.

The Civil Ombudsman deals with 20–40 complaints a year concerning health services. These complaints represent 2–3% of the cases reviewed by the Ombudsman. Taking into consideration the importance of the health service within public administration as a whole, the Ombudsman plays a relatively minor role in securing the rule of law for patients.

The Patient Ombudsman ('the Ombudsman')

The first official record of proposals to have a special Patient Ombudsman dates from 1975. In a report to Parliament about 'The Rule of Law in Social and Health Institutions' the Ministry of Social Affairs discussed, *inter alia*, whether patients in such institutions should have a special Ombudsman to whom they may present their complaint. The background to this was partly the special needs that patients in such institutions were deemed to have. It was also partly the experience that such patients did not tend to complain to the Civil Ombudsman or other official control bodies. Five years later, in the context of preparing a new law relating to medical practitioners, the issue of a Patient Ombudsman was raised again. Again the conclusion was that there was no need for such a specific Ombudsman.

During the 1980s patients' rights developed into a central concept within Norwegian legal research, public debate, health administration and the administration of justice. The concept of patients' rights had particularly positive connotations, and was accorded considerable weight in health politics. A part of this development was that most of the counties during the second part of the 1980s and the 1990s established Patient Ombudsman schemes. This meant that the counties, at this time responsible for secondary healthcare, including all hospitals, set up Ombudsman schemes on a 'volunteer' basis that had secondary health services as their function.

The Patient Ombudsmen were through county directives afforded a relatively free professional position. They could not in specific cases be influenced by, for example, the county administration or hospital directors. At the end of the 1990s the Patient Ombudsmen annually received about 5000 requests which they investigated. In the county and municipality of Oslo a special Ombudsman scheme was arranged. In addition to secondary health services, this scheme also included primary care and social services.

Within this framework Patient Ombudsman schemes involved different functions depending on the county. Some of the Ombudsmen took on the role of 'reporter', 'spokesman' or even 'lawyer'; some acted as 'intermediaries'; some more like a 'spiritual adviser'; and others again acted as 'jacks-of-all-trades'!

Some of the first Patient Ombudsmen also struggled to be accepted. Articles by physicians presented in the *Journal of the Norwegian Medical Association* and in the newspapers showed that parts of the medical system feared that the Ombudsmen would exacerbate disputes and conflicts rather than resolve them.

During the late 1980s and the 1990s some of the Patient Ombudsman schemes were evaluated. Some articles related to this new institution were also published. In one of these the following opinion on the future of the system, based on experiences documented until that time, was set out:

> The aim with the Patient Ombudsman must be to safeguard the patient's interest and legal rights and be a suitable measure to improve the quality of the healthcare services. ... The scheme must in the future (also)
>
> - be regulated by law
> - have health services as a whole as their function
> - be free of charge
> - be organised regionally
> - carry out the work independently
> - have legal competence.[9]

At the end of the 1990s nearly all counties had their own Patient Ombudsman. From 2001 the Patient Ombudsman institution is statutory in each county. In the following, the term Patient Ombudsman will be used when referring to both the institution itself and to the staff at each Ombudsman office. The context of the text will clarify if it is the institution or the Ombudsman staff that is being referred to.

Summary

During the 1980s and 1990s patients' rights developed into a central concept in Norwegian health legislation. At the same time several complaint procedures and investigative bodies were established to which patients could turn when they wanted to have a case reviewed or when they were dissatisfied. The Patient Ombudsman is the most important of these institutions. The Civil Ombudsman receives only a few complaints from patients: between 20 and 40 per year. In the year 2000 the Civil Ombudsman received 38, equivalent to 3% of all cases. Moreover, the Civil Ombudsman only raised two cases on his own initiative. At the same time the 19 Patient Ombudsmen received several thousand cases, which makes the Patient Ombudsman the more important to users of health services.

The organisational structure of Patient Ombudsmen

Legal basis

The Patient Ombudsman scheme is based upon the Act on Patients' Rights. The purpose, scope and powers are outlined in chapter 8 of the law. The scheme is described in more detail in the proposition presented by the ministry to Parliament (Odelsting) and in the recommendation from the health committee to Parliament.[10,11] The Ministry of Health is empowered to issue regulations, but such regulations have not yet been provided.

Level of functions

Until 2001 Patient Ombudsmen were established on a regional level. Each of the counties themselves organised their own Ombudsman. From 2002 the 19 Patient Ombudsmen have become a national institution. This is linked to the fact that the state is now the principal provider of secondary care. The government is responsible for ensuring this, within the confines of § 8-2: 'Every county municipality shall have a patient ombud.' Each Patient Ombudsman therefore still has the county as his geographical jurisdiction. People who either live or receive health services in a particular county may use the Ombudsman located in that county.

The Patient Ombudsman and the Civil Ombudsman thus have different principles and somewhat different areas of jurisdiction. The Civil Ombudsman answers to Parliament, its office is located in Oslo, and it has the whole country as its jurisdiction. The Patient Ombudsmen on the other hand answer to the Ministry of Health, are located in each county and have their attention focused on health services and the local population.

Localisation and staffing

Usually the Patient Ombudsman has an office located in one of the larger cities in the county, often next to where the largest hospital is situated. The staff working at the office of the Patient Ombudsman have no other functions, which avoids potential conflicts of interest. The level of staffing in the Patient Ombudsman offices ranges from 1 to 10. Oslo has the biggest office, the reason being that the Oslo office also has primary healthcare and social services as part of its responsibilities. Usually the Patient Ombudsman is a lawyer but in some cases they might be health professionals with legal training. It is common that the staff working at the bigger Ombudsman offices collectively have dual competence.

Funding arrangements

The funding for the Patient Ombudsman is provided by the state. The state also decides on the staffing level for each Ombudsman office. There is no fixed norm for this. In practice the state has taken over employment of the staff that were originally appointed in each county. The Patient Ombudsman is intended as a free service for every citizen and does not levy any charges.

Regulation and accountability

The law sets out the framework for further regulation. In § 8-2 it is stated 'The ombud shall carry out his work independently'. This means that the Ombudsman shall discharge his duties autonomously and independently of the ministry and other public institutions. Parliament emphasised this in their comments on the provision. So it is clear that no one can influence the Ombudsman in individual cases.

§ 8-8 states 'The ministry may issue regulations on the implementation of the provisions relating to the patient ombud and may also issue supplements to these provisions'. This provision has to be seen in the light of § 8-2. Regulations and guidelines may thus be issued for example regarding organisational and administrative questions, such as staffing and training demands. Such provisions have not yet been published. It is likely that provisions will be issued later, as the system is still undergoing the transition from administration by the counties to the state.

Discussion

In many ways the organisational structure is fixed. There is a legal basis for the scheme, there is clarity about the level of functions, the funding arrangements are clear and there is no doubt that the Ombudsman works independently. There may, however, in the future be a challenge to the independence of the Ombudsman in that the system is organised under the Ministry of Health as this body is now also responsible for and organises the delivery of secondary healthcare. However, since it is so clearly stipulated in law and 'travaux préparatoires'[10,11] that the Ombudsman shall work independently, there should be no reason to fear that public authorities will try to influence the decisions and actions made by the Patient Ombudsman. In future, however, it may be important to introduce greater legal competence, since the work is inextricably linked to patients' rights.

Role and functions

Aims

The objective of the Patient Ombudsman scheme is twofold; first, it concerns the interests of the individual patient. Second, it is about the general quality of healthcare. As stated in § 8-2: 'The patient ombud shall work to safeguard patients' rights, interests and legal rights in their relations with the health service and to improve the quality of the health service.' Consequently, the Ombudsman is regarded as an important institution in regard to improving quality and applying the rule of law in the health services.

Parliament has emphasised that the Patient Ombudsman should act in different ways to achieve this aim. The Ombudsman should pursue cases following complaints from patients/citizens. He should also on his own initiative pursue cases that in other ways come to his knowledge, and should be pro-active in seeking such intelligence. It is expected that the Ombudsman should also feed this knowledge back to the health service.

According to § 8-1 the Ombudsman shall work with 'legal rights' as well as patients' needs and interests from a general perspective.[11] The focus should be both on the individual patient and on patients as a group.[12] In terms of needs and interests, it is said that the Ombudsman should make contact and communicate with the health service to feed back what patients have experienced and what they think, and thus also seek to avert more formal conflict. As to legal rights, the Ombudsman should be an intermediary for complaints to the right places. The Ombudsman determines together with the patient to whom the complaint should be directed depending on its nature, for example to the County Medical Officer or the patient compensation scheme.

Functions

The functions of the Patient Ombudsman involve, according to § 8-2, public secondary healthcare only. This means that the Ombudsman shall not deal with private specialist health services (a rather small sector), nor with primary health-care. Patients not satisfied with these elements of health services may, however, get information from the Ombudsman on how to make a complaint. Usually the County Medical Officer is appropriate for such complaints as there is no informal route like the Patient Ombudsman for dealing with such cases.

In legal matters the Ombudsman will have to deal regularly with cases relating to the Act on Patients' Rights, the Act on Specialised Health Services, the Act on Mental Health Care and the Act on Health Personnel. All these acts apply in terms of secondary healthcare. The question is on the one hand if patients' rights have been violated and on the other hand if the health service and/or health staff have fulfilled their duties. In some cases the question also arises as to whether patients are entitled to compensation under the Act on Patient Compensation.

Tasks

When a patient asks the Patient Ombudsman for assistance, it follows from § 8-7(1) that 'To a reasonable extent, the patient ombud shall give anyone who requests it information, advice and guidance in matters that are included in the work of the ombud'. The focus is on advice and guidance. This means that the central task involves giving patients information about rights and duties, and about the next step in the complaint procedure. However, the service also includes, for example, supporting patients if they have not understood what has happened or will happen in the course of their treatment, or need to meet with health service staff. It also involves handling complaints either informally by asking health services to perform their duties towards the patient, or more formally where the County Medical Officer is asked to reverse a decision and/or to discipline a member of staff or an institution.

The Patient Ombudsman has the right to make his opinion public. As stated in § 8-7 subsection two, 'The patient ombud is entitled to give his opinion on matters that are included in the work of the ombud, and to suggest concrete measures of improvement. The patient ombud himself shall decide to whom these statements shall be directed.' This power supports the Ombudsman's role as an important body in introducing solutions and improvements. He may give an opinion in cases relating to both individual patients and groups.

The Ombudsman may not, however, do anything against the will of the patient. If a patient does not wish to make a complaint to the County Medical Officer, the Ombudsman must respect this, even if it is obvious that the patient would win his or her case. If it is important to highlight the problems raised by the case as a point of principle, the Ombudsman may use the case anonymously.

When a case is closed, the Ombudsman must inform the patient of the outcome, and explain the reasons for this. As stated in § 8-8 subsection three 'The patient ombud shall notify anyone who has made a request to the ombud of the outcome following the handling of a case, and a brief explanation of the result'. This may also include, depending on circumstances, forwarding a copy of the final report from the Ombudsman to the relevant health body, or a copy of the complaint to the County Medical Officer. It may also include a copy of the hospital's final report to the Ombudsman about any complications in connection with treatment, linked to any conclusion by the Patient Ombudsman that there is no legal justification for claiming compensation.

In the preparatory work of the law it is explicitly stated that the Ombudsman may present suggestions for quality improvement and should also be actively involved by the hospitals in their work for achieving this.

In some situations the Ombudsman has a duty to inform the supervisory authority (in practice the County Medical Officer) about a case. From § 8-7 subsection four it follows that 'The patient ombud shall notify the supervising authorities of conditions where a follow-up by the authorities is required.' However, it is not clear when such action is required. In practice the supervisory authority always follows up cases involving suspected negligent breach of duty by health services or health personnel, which have resulted in a considerable burden to the patient or represent a threat to the safety of health services. If the Patient Ombudsman has knowledge of such a situation, he probably has a duty to report this to the County Medical Officer regardless of the opinion of the patient involved.

Power

The Patient Ombudsman does not make material decisions that are binding for others. As mentioned the Ombudsman makes statements, but according to § 8-7 subsection two these statements 'are not mandatory'. They have only the weight that health staff or services choose to give them. This depends very much on the real impact of the statements, how convincing they are in terms of substance and argument, and the general credibility the Ombudsman has built up through previous investigations.

If the Patient Ombudsman and the hospital do not share the same opinion on a legal question, the Ombudsman may, according to § 8-7, bring the case to the County Medical Officer for a legally binding decision. The County Medical Officer has the power to interpret the law and make such a decision. In practice the threat of action before the County Medical Officer often leads to an agreement with the hospital.

If the patient seeks compensation the case must be brought before the patient compensation scheme to be reviewed. Frequently the Patient Ombudsman gets involved in cases about injuries potentially linked to treatment in hospitals. In such cases the Ombudsman may first ask for information to clarify the facts. Hospitals are obliged to answer these requests (*see* p. 103), and to send a copy of the record. Having reviewed the case, the Ombudsman helps the patient to contact the patient compensation scheme.

Discussion

There are two main aims with the Patient Ombudsman scheme: to safeguard patients' interests and legal rights; and to contribute to the quality of the health services. The first role is probably seen as the most important. As patients' interests concentrate on legal rights because of the Act on Patient Rights, the Ombudsman's role must be focused on how these rights are being met. The second aim could be seen as deriving from the first. The Patient Ombudsman should use the experience drawn from individual cases to compile reports to send back to the hospital.

The Patient Ombudsman's function is limited to secondary healthcare. Parliament has not provided any clear reasoning for this limitation. It has been suggested that patients more often have problems linked to hospitals than to primary healthcare. Experience also shows that hospital services more often result in bad outcomes where patients need support. This is a limitation that has not been debated extensively. A group within Parliament has therefore recently asked the ministry to present a paper discussing this matter.

The legislature has not accorded the Patient Ombudsman the same levels of formal authority as for example the Civil Ombudsman (*see* p. 96). It is therefore not predetermined that health service institutions will comply with statements from the Patient Ombudsman, which perhaps is why this Ombudsman is more reserved in issuing statements.

Case-handling – the law

The right to contact the Patient Ombudsman

Everyone has the right to contact the Patient Ombudsman about matters concerning public secondary healthcare services; *see* § 8-3(2): 'Anyone may contact the patient ombud and request that a case be handled.' The provision includes two important points. The first is that, in addition to patients (and their relatives), anyone may contact the Ombudsman to have a case handled. The second point is that their requests are not named as complaints, however, only as requests that should be handled by the Ombudsman under the perspective of safeguarding patients' rights, interests and legal rights and of improving the health services.

Healthcare staff and health services themselves may thus use the Patient Ombudsman to have cases investigated as well as patients. However, if the case relates to a particular patient, only that patient can decide what involvement the Ombudsman should have.

It is not necessary to make a formal request when contacting the Ombudsman. As stated in § 8-3, handling may either be on the basis of an oral request or a written request. This is a part of the concept that there should be a low threshold for accessing the Ombudsman.

The right to confidentiality

Usually the patients or other individuals who contact the Patient Ombudsman reveal their identity. According to § 8-3(2) 'Persons who contact the patient ombud are entitled to be anonymous'. This means that the Patient Ombudsman may not ask individuals giving information to disclose their identity. In practice, anonymous health professionals provide information, for example about an action which they consider has been to the detriment of a patient or patients as a group and should be remedied. The Ombudsman has to respect anonymity, but this may create more difficulties in investigating a case. If the information given relates to an identified patient, this patient has the right to decide what kind of support he should have or what should be done.

Handling of the requests

The Patient Ombudsman is not obliged to handle every case presented. As stated in § 8-4 'The patient ombud shall by himself determine if a request provides adequate grounds for further handling'. Then it will depend on the priorities of the Ombudsman whether the case is followed up. It is presumed, however, that the Ombudsman will normally take the case. If this does not happen, it is stated in § 8-4 that 'the person who made the request shall be notified thereof, and be given a brief explanation for this decision'. The explanation must be in written form if the person bringing the case to the Ombudsman is not anonymous. One reason for not handling the case may be that the Ombudsman considers it to relate to a part of the health service that falls outside his jurisdiction. Another reason may be that the patient is not satisfied with the conclusion of the investigation carried out by the Ombudsman.

The Patient Ombudsman has the right to obtain information. According to § 8-5 'Public authorities and other bodies that provide services for the public administration shall give the ombud the required information in order for the ombud to carry out his tasks'. This means that any such authority shall give information, not only bodies within the secondary healthcare services. So a doctor in primary care must likewise provide the Ombudsman with the information requested. This might be about treatment, communication, correspondence etc. There are few limitations to this right to demand information, though the provisions of the Civil Procedure Act § 204–209 (about confidentiality) apply correspondingly to the Patient Ombudsman.

In the course of investigating a case, the Patient Ombudsman shall also have access to all premises where public health services are being provided. While the right to obtain information applies to all public authorities, access to the premises applies only to secondary healthcare services. This limitation does not in practice present problems as primary care is outside the Ombudsman's field of work.

Bringing cases to a close

As mentioned above (*see* p. 96), the Civil Ombudsman shall render a decision on all cases proceeding from a complaint or which have been taken up on his own initiative. By 'decision' is meant a statement about the outcome. The Patient Ombudsman is not obliged to make such a statement. The decision can take different forms and the case may end by not taking any decision at all. Thus, the Patient Ombudsman does not have to close cases in specific ways. The reason for this is that in many cases it is not appropriate for the Patient Ombudsman to make statements. The expectation is often that the Ombudsman instead sets cases on the right decision-making track. If for example the Patient Ombudsman considers that a health service provider is not respecting the law in spite of what he has said, he may, with permission from the patient, bring the case as a complaint to the County Medical Officer who has the power to adjudicate the matter.

Publicity and periodic reporting

According to the Act relating to Patients' Rights (§ 8-7) the Patient Ombudsmen have the duty to publicise their own decision-making. They achieve such publicity in different ways. Frequently the newspapers have articles about the Ombudsmen in general and linked to special cases they have handled.

At the end of the year each of the Patient Ombudsmen publishes an annual report about activity and results. The reports are open to public review and it is common that the newspapers refer to these reports. In this way the Ombudsmen also get publicity not only about individual cases that patients wish to have aired, but also about their activity in general. Starting in 2003 data from all individual cases will be registered in the same way and collected in a shared register. Consequently we will have aggregated data from all regional Ombudsmen.

Discussion

It should be easy to contact the Patient Ombudsman: and this is clear, in particular, from the fact that anyone may make an oral request. On the other hand, it is the Ombudsman who determines whether a request provides adequate grounds for further investigation. In reality, therefore, the Ombudsman has a good deal of control over individual cases.

Often, different courses of action are taken depending on what the Patient Ombudsman considers appropriate in any given case. The role he sees himself playing, or the role he has competence to play, may influence these decisions, and the result for the patient. Whether the Ombudsman sees himself on the one hand as a lawyer or on the other as a spiritual adviser will in individual cases often have a significant impact on the handling of the case. If the patient is dissatisfied with the work done by the Patient Ombudsman, he or she may appeal to the Civil Ombudsman, but in practice such cases have yet to be raised. This may indicate that patients are seldom very dissatisfied with the case-handling.

Case-handling – the practice

As mentioned above, there has been a shift in the system since 2001. From that point Patient Ombudsmen operated under the Act on Patients' Rights, and since 2002 they worked under the aegis of the state. There has not been any evaluation of the Patient Ombudsman scheme following these changes. However, in reality there have been few changes to practice, and observations about practice in the 1990s will therefore to a great extent also be valid today.

To illustrate case-handling in practice, a helpful starting point is to use data from the annual reports given by the Patient Ombudsmen and evaluations that have been carried through. There has been no common evaluation of the different arrangements, but some of them have been evaluated individually. For the purposes of this chapter, the Patient Ombudsman selected is in the county of Nordland. This is in several respects an average Norwegian county, the arrangement there has lasted for many years and it has been evaluated twice, most recently in 1997.[13] This will be supplemented by data from some of the other Ombudsmen.

Availability

Of the 308 patients surveyed during the evaluation of the Patient Ombudsman in the county of Nordland, 92% answered that it had been easy to contact the Ombudsman. Data from other counties confirm this. In contacting the Ombudsman, 50% in Nordland said that they used the telephone, 20% that they wrote a letter, and 16% that they met the Ombudsman while he was visiting the hospital. The remainder were unsure which method was used first.

Enquiries and cases

The Patient Ombudsman in Nordland receives about 750 enquiries a year from patients and others. Compared with other Patient Ombudsmen this is a comparatively high figure. From this, the Ombudsman investigates about 200 cases a year linked to specialist health services (a similar level to that of the 1990s).

Of the 308 cases raised by the patients that took part in the evaluation in Nordland, females represented around 55%. People older than 50 raised about half of the cases. Patients themselves raised about 75% of cases, relatives approximately 20%, and others around 5% of the cases. This breakdown has remained largely the same for the last 10 years.

According to the annual reports, there is reason to believe that Patient Ombudsmen nationwide receive more than 10 000 enquiries and that about 5000 requests are investigated as cases. These figures seem to have stabilised in the last two years, owing to the fact that all counties have now been through an initial start-up period. Figures are not expected to change much in the future. However, whether the individual Ombudsman investigates an enquiry, the approach taken and follow up vary. For example one Ombudsman one year undertook only 12 investigations out of 365 enquiries.

The Ombudsman in Oslo also deals with cases from social services and primary care in addition to secondary healthcare services. In the year 2000, 500 cases were investigated related to primary care, 1740 connected to social services and 490 cases linked to secondary healthcare services. This indicates that patients are seeking assistance just as much in primary care as in connection with secondary health-care. The need for assistance may possibly differ outside Oslo, but there are no specific reasons to think so. Nevertheless, this system should be evaluated, perhaps by a project where the Ombudsman in a county like Nordland has his functions extended to cover primary healthcare.

Why do patients contact the Patient Ombudsman?

The 308 individuals in Nordland who had chosen to contact the Ombudsman gave the following reasons for this (many gave more than one reason) (Table 6.1).

Table 6.1 Reasons for contacting the Ombudsman

Reason	Number	Percentage
To complain about possible bad treatment	232	33
To obtain more treatment/another examination	107	15
To obtain more information	62	9
To have (copy of) my own record	49	7
To complain about rude behaviour	131	19
To complain about routines etc in the hospital	86	12
Other	33	5
Total	700	100

From these figures it seems that many patients contact the Patient Ombudsman for medical reasons or reasons closely linked to medicine. Some 50% complain about not receiving the expected examination/treatment or about failure of treat-ment. The Patient Ombudsman registers the reasons linked to various cases, but only registers the primary ground for the request. About 80% of these cases are linked to treatment: the need for examination or further/another treatment, or more usually complaints about possible failures and faults, especially linked to injury. This breakdown seems to apply similarly for many other Patient Ombudsmen.

The same 308 individuals also reported what they wanted to achieve through their contact with the Ombudsman. Many of them gave more than one reason. Their answers are summarised in Table 6.2.

The data tell us that it is important for patients that health professionals communicate openly about what has happened in connection with their treatment. It is fair to say that the patients want primarily to be listened to and be given a positive acknowledgement of what they have experienced.

Assistance

Of the 308 patients mentioned above about 75% said that the time taken for the Patient Ombudsman to finish an investigation was not too long. Some 60% were

Table 6.2   What people want from the Ombudsman

Reason	Number	Percentage
To get advice	124	17
To get help having their case clarified	171	23
To obtain compensation	87	12
To get an admission of fault	139	19
To prevent others encountering the same situation	118	16
To get new examination/treatment	92	12
Other	11	1
Total	742	100

more satisfied than dissatisfied with the help that they had received from the Ombudsman. Likewise slightly more than 60% considered that their case had been sufficiently analysed. However, about 40% felt that the Ombudsman showed unduly more consideration for the hospital and the health personnel.

In another evaluation in the county of Nordland 68% said that the Ombudsman had been of great support, 24% that it had been of some support, while only 8% said that the assistance given had been of little or no help.

Evaluations were also carried out in other counties through the 1990s. They have yielded more or less the same results, though some have been more favourable to the Patient Ombudsman. Indeed, no evaluations were such as to recommend finishing the existing Ombudsman arrangement or special measures to change it in a radical way. When the ministry summarised countrywide experience of the Patient Ombudsmen towards the end of the 1990s, the fact that most patients seemed to be satisfied with their work was emphasised.[10]

Some cases in Nordland each year are taken on to institutions outside secondary healthcare to reach a final solution or decision. Some 20–25% of the investigated cases were taken to the patient compensation scheme, and another 10% were put to the County Medical Officer. These figures vary for the various Patient Ombudsmen, depending on their interpretation of the role of Ombudsman. Ombudsmen with legal training, such as the Patient Ombudsman in Nordland, tend to support patients well on legal matters, while others partly may (feel they) lack competence to do so and more often recommend the patient to seek specialist legal advice.

The effect of the Ombudsman's intervention

There are no general data describing in detail the effect of the Ombudsmen. However, separate evaluations indicate that the Ombudsmen play an important role. Patients have to a great extent obtained further examinations, further treatment, more information, copies of their records, and compensation and ex gratia payments they would otherwise not have obtained.[14] For example an evaluation from the State University Hospital concluded that over a two-year period 90 patients at that hospital had received a total of 2 million USD that they probably would not have been paid had they not contacted the Patient Ombudsman.[9]

In Nordland 226 health personnel engaged in secondary healthcare services answered some questions about their opinion of the Patient Ombudsman scheme. First they were asked to relate what effect they thought the Ombudsman had on themselves and on the hospital. Of the 226 respondents some 50% said this was a necessary supplement to the existing safeguard measures, while 10% said they considered it unnecessary to have an Ombudsman. Nearly half the group said that the existence of the Ombudsman made it more important for them to exercise internal professional controls than had been the case before. Likewise nearly 60% said that the internal control routines in the hospital had become more important.

These health personnel were also asked to evaluate what effect they thought the Ombudsman scheme had had in general (not just their specific experience in Nordland), in terms of supporting patients' interests and legal rights. As many as 87% said that this was important/very important, while only 13% considered it not very important. It appears that health personnel consider the Patient Ombudsman scheme to be positive and have the view that it is an important factor in safeguarding patients' interests and legal rights.

Co-operation between the Patient Ombudsmen

The 19 Patient Ombudsmen work in a decentralised way. Some of them work alone, and to some extent they have different professional qualifications. They (therefore) tend to choose different roles and use different methods. To respond to this problem, Patient Ombudsmen arrange annual meetings to exchange experiences and discuss working methods, which are organised on their own initiative. Some Ombudsmen meet regionally a few times a year to assist each other in resolving difficulties. Many of the Patient Ombudsmen consider these meetings important and provide new input into their daily work. In addition to the web-site of each Patient Ombudsman they have a common web-site. This co-operation process will probably, and hopefully, develop as the state has now taken over responsibility for the Patient Ombudsman scheme. For example the Ombudsmen currently have no elected body representing them when problems emerge that are shared.

Discussion

It is seen as easy for patients to contact the Patient Ombudsmen. In practice many do get in touch with them. The caseload of the Patient Ombudsmen concerns mainly medical problems, in particular complaints about bad outcomes or injuries sustained. Procedural questions play a minor role.

Most patients are satisfied with the help they get from the Patient Ombudsmen. However, a number seem not to be. This may be linked to the fact that the Ombudsman may not fulfil his functions properly. Some of the Patient Ombudsmen work alone and do not get the supervision they may need. Likewise the personalities involved and their professional skills may vary, but these are very important for the level of help a patient gets. Another reason for dissatisfaction may be that many patients have unrealistic expectations about what can be done. The experience of County Medical Officers handling complaints is also that patients often have such expectations and only one-third are successful in their action.

Health personnel regard the Patient Ombudsman scheme as an important safe-guard for patients although it is not clear why this is the case. Health personnel may also fear that the Patient Ombudsman will create extra burdens or even create trouble for them without grounds.

It is important for patients to know that they have someone in a formal position to contact when they need assistance. In the end it is practical results that count for the most. Evidence from specific evaluation exercises and studies indicates that the Ombudsman scheme provides a substantial benefit that patients would not have obtained without the Ombudsman's intervention.

The Patient Ombudsman in Nordland, like many others of the Ombudsmen, has several times addressed general concerns to the hospitals. We do not know in detail from written material what kind of results this or other more general activities of the Ombudsmen have achieved. However, there are many statements in the annual reports indicating that the Ombudsmen have played an important role in changing systems to ensure the quality of health services. Some of the Ombudsmen also participate in the hospitals' quality committee meetings.

Analysis

Every year thousands of patients approach their Patient Ombudsman seeking assistance. The Ombudsman co-operates with hospitals and other bodies to promote patients' interests and their legitimate demands. This institution is now generally well accepted by hospital administrators, physicians and nurses. It is for example seldom that Ombudsmen do not receive replies in due time when investigating cases. It is arguable that the Patient Ombudsmen now hold a relatively strong position in local communities, and in this respect have benefited to some extent from the already established reputation of the Civil Ombudsman. Likewise there is reason to believe that the Ombudsmen have benefited from the position that cases brought to them seldom find their way to the courts. Since any cases involving injury to patients tend to end up within the patient compensation scheme this represents far less of a confrontational approach for the health professionals.

Set out in the introduction above are some basic elements that 10 years ago (five years after the first Patient Ombudsmen schemes started) were considered necessary for a well-functioning Patient Ombudsman scheme. Some of these elements have now been put into practice: the Patient Ombudsman scheme is regulated by law and is organised regionally; help is free of charge; the Patient Ombudsman carries out his work independently and has no other role besides working as an Ombudsman. Some elements are not fulfilled, though: the Patient Ombudsman still has only the specific remit of secondary healthcare services, and there is no regulation conferring *legal* competence on him. The issue now is whether it is time to enlarge the scheme to include primary healthcare. Experience from Oslo supports this: in fact more patients seek assistance about primary care than secondary care. The general trend in recent years in Norway is to use legislation more in underpinning patients' interests. This legislative expansion supports the position that the Ombudsman should be required to have undertaken legal training. This would probably also strengthen the Ombudsman's authority in many of the cases handled.

Today the Patient Ombudsmen in different counties undertake various roles. This may follow on from the local guidelines given. In theory these do not differ significantly, and many of the variations appear quite abstract. Information and evaluation exercises from the late 1990s tell us that the Patient Ombudsmen themselves have differing attitudes towards their role which may explain the variations in practice. Some state that they act more as lawyers, some as intermediaries, some as spiritual advisers, and some state that they mix these roles.

The role of the Patient Ombudsman should be developed. They need at the very least an organisational body or a forum that can develop and shape their future role. Though it is important that the ombudsmen in their action allow for the local conditions that may differ a lot, we should be able to expect that every Patient Ombudsman will generally take almost the same action in the same situation. Some functions are common to all systems today, but some Ombudsmen will more than likely have to modify their practice to come into line with a more 'standard practice'.

- The Patient Ombudsman should first offer informal support, to ensure that the problem is dealt with by the relevant health service provider.
- If the service provider does not want to take action in relation to examination or treatment, the Patient Ombudsman should pursue the matter, and seek further information if the patient is dissatisfied with the answer given by the service provider.
- If the Ombudsman is of the opinion that the service provider is breaking the law, this should be made explicit. Ultimately, the Ombudsman should help patients to complain to the County Medical Officer.
- If the health service provider does not wish to take action in a case of potential injury, the Patient Ombudsman should ask the service provider for more information about the damage and additionally seek a copy of the relevant medical records. It must be a part of his role to help the patient pursue a claim for damages with the patient compensation scheme if a compensation award may be appropriate.

Over time the Patient Ombudsman will collect information accumulated from individual case investigations, which should be of great interest to hospitals, and ultimately to specific units in hospitals. It is important that the Ombudsmen can identify problems that recur and try to ensure that the health service providers take action to deal with such problems. We note that some Ombudsmen, on the basis of experience, alone or together with representatives from hospitals, initiate and also participate in studies that seek to investigate and understand such problems and try to identify the measures needed as a result.

The knowledge and the information the Patient Ombudsmen obtain are highly relevant to the education of other healthcare workers. It is a role for many of the Patient Ombudsmen in practice to pass on their knowledge and experience to, for example, groups of health staff. This must be seen in connection with the problem that some health personnel do on occasion seek to avoid their duty to inform patients about their right to contact the Ombudsman. As a part of this educational activity the Ombudsman can underline the fact that it is the health staff themselves who have the principal duty to protect patients' rights and inform patients of these rights.

From this it can be said that the primary function of the Patient Ombudsmen is not really to deal with resolving dissatisfaction. Nor should they generally act as a spiritual adviser. It is also clear enough that they should not act as 'jacks-of-all-trades'.

The role should be mainly linked to patients' rights and to improving quality. In the community the focus is frequently on whether the Ombudsman should act as 'a lawyer or a bridge-builder'. These can, however, often be seen as two sides of the same coin: either acting formally or informally. The answer is therefore not an 'either-or'. The focus should be on using an informal approach initially, and if this line does not achieve results, then formal steps can be taken.

It may be a constant challenge to a Patient Ombudsman to meet different patients, health personnel and representatives and to find solutions acceptable to everyone. Bridge-building presupposes not only a specific attitude, but also personal skill. The Ombudsman needs legal knowledge, and training to enable him to operate as a negotiator. Individual qualities such as the ability to listen to other people, communication and conciliation skills are also important. Taken altogether, Ombudsmen need a good deal of training to live up to the exacting requirements of this package of demands.

The Patient Ombudsman scheme has developed over a period of 15 years. It is well known among patients, and has a generally good reputation across the community. The Ombudsman is easy to contact, provides important assistance to patients, and is seen as a significant part of the system for ensuring that patients avail themselves of their rights and that the quality of the health services is improved. The Ombudsman has a clear position among the health institutions, and has an important role in achieving solutions for patients in need of a mediator or a spokesperson. A significant part of the Ombudsman's role must also be to emphasise and resort to legal measures when other approaches are inappropriate or have failed.

The Patient Ombudsmen's role is not only linked to giving assistance to the individual patient. They shall, according to the law, also work to improve the quality of health services. It is not really possible at this stage to measure the true impact of their activities. However, as the Ombudsmen regularly take a systematic approach in their dealings with hospitals, present more general concerns to the hospitals, and in addition sometimes are asked to be involved by the hospitals in their quality improvement activities, it appears that the Ombudsmen probably do to some extent contribute to this. As the Patient Ombudsmen have become units under the same administrative system starting in 2002, it will perhaps be easier in future to develop their activities in accordance with this greater objective.

Since 2001 we have introduced new legislation that gives patients increased rights, especially within secondary healthcare services. Likewise there are provisions giving patients new rights to make complaints and have health service decisions reversed. It is too early to say what kind of impact this will have on the Patient Ombudsmen's operations. It is however expected that in the future they will have more of a role in legal matters as patients begin increasingly to use their rights and have their cases heard. Also in the future the Patient Ombudsmen should take on the role of bridge-builder. When this route fails or is not appropriate, the Ombudsmen must act much more as lawyers, arguing the point or bringing the case to the right public forum, such as the County Medical Officer and/or the patient compensation scheme. A challenge to the Ombudsmen is to develop further procedures for co-operating with these institutions, while not forgetting their second main role – that is to contribute to the improvement of the quality of the health services.

Another category of challenge to the Ombudsmen would be if the Ministry of Health as administrator started to regulate and manage their activity in many ways. That should not happen.

Conclusions and recommendations

Complaints from patients can be submitted at the level of the medical institution where healthcare is delivered (the municipalities, the healthcare enterprises). If patients believe that their legal rights have been violated, they may also complain to the County Medical Officer. The County Medical Officer has the power to reverse a decision made by the medical institutions and also to discipline health personnel and institutions. If patients believe they are entitled to compensation, they may make requests to the patient compensation scheme. Patients who think they need assistance from others to have their needs, interests and legal rights met by healthcare providers (in secondary health services), or need assistance contacting or presenting a case before the County Medical Officer or the patient compensation scheme, may seek and get such assistance from the Patient Ombudsman.

From our experience in Norway through 15 years of what has worked well and not so well, it seems appropriate to conclude with the following recommendations:

- the scheme must have its basis in law
- the scheme must be publicly financed and be free of charge
- the scheme must be locally organised
- the role of the Patient Ombudsman must be clarified and sufficiently publicised
- the Patient Ombudsman must work independently
- the Patient Ombudsman must have the authority to investigate cases
- the Patient Ombudsman must help patients to avail themselves of their legal rights
- the Patient Ombudsman must primarily work in an informal way
- the Patient Ombudsman must, if necessary, use the formal system to assist patients
- the Patient Ombudsman must give a written reason for not handling cases
- the Patient Ombudsman (staff) should have both legal and health competence
- the Patient Ombudsman must not at the same time work in any other role
- the Patient Ombudsmen should co-operate between themselves and have a professional forum for doing so
- the Patient Ombudsmen should aggregate data from the requests and investigations and use these data in their contact with hospitals and health authorities to contribute to the improvement of health services
- the Patient Ombudsmen must also report their activities to the public
- the scheme must be regularly evaluated.

The time has probably now come for the Patient Ombudsmen in Norway to also have as their mandate in general terms the role of safeguarding the interests and the legal rights of patients in relation to the primary healthcare services. The Ministry of Health, being responsible for the delivery of specialised health services, should also consider carefully whether this Ministry would be the right one to, and how they should, administrate the Patient Ombudsman scheme. There are possible conflicting interests.

References

1   Kjønstad A (1999) The development of patients' rights in Norway. In: O Molven (ed.) *The Norwegian Health Care System. Legal and Organizational Aspects.* University of Oslo, Oslo.

2   Molven O (2002) The guiding principles of Norwegian health legislation. In: O Molven (ed.) *Health Legislation in Norway.* Ad notam, Oslo.

3   Kjønstad A (2002) Rights of citizens to primary health care. In: O Molven (ed.) *Health Legislation in Norway.* Ad notam, Oslo.

4   Kjønstad A (2002) The right to hospital services and other specialised health care. In: O Molven (ed.) *Health Legislation in Norway.* Ad notam, Oslo.

5   Kjønstad A (2002) The rights of patients in Norway. In: O Molven (ed.) *Health Legislation in Norway.* Ad notam, Oslo.

6   Shetelig AW (1999) Supervising the national health care services. In: O Molven (ed.) *The Norwegian Health Care System. Legal and Organisational Aspects.* University of Oslo, Oslo.

7   Molven O (2002) Reactions against health personnel that are not complying with the law. In: O Molven (ed.) *Health Legislation in Norway.* Ad notam, Oslo.

8   Reiersen N (2002) Compensation to patients after injury. In: O Molven (ed.) *Health Legislation in Norway.* Ad notam, Oslo.

9   Molven O (1991) The Patient Ombudsman Scheme: a contribution to legal safeguards and quality in the health service? *Lov og Rett (Norwegian Law Journal).* 195–222. (Only in Norwegian.)

10   Proposition No. 12 (1998–99) to the Odelsting (Parliament). About the Act on Patients' Rights, Chapter 8. (Only in Norwegian.)

11   Recommendation No. 91 (1998–99) to the Odelsting (Parliament). About the Act on Patients' Rights. (Only in Norwegian.)

12   Segest E (1997) The Ombudsman's involvement in ensuring patients' rights. *Medicine and Law.* **16**(3): 473–86.

13   HBO Report 7/1997. *'Advocate or bridge builder'. Evaluation of the Nordland Patient Ombudsman Scheme.* (Only in Norwegian.)

14   Molven O (1989) Patient Ombudsman at the State University Hospital. Experience with a 2-year trial. *Tidsskr Nor Laegeforening (The Journal of the Norwegian Medical Association).* **109**(24): 2457–60. (English summary.)

CHAPTER 7

The British Health Service Ombudsman

Philip Giddings

Introduction – the geopolitical position in Britain

The United Kingdom is a parliamentary democracy, a unitary state, with elected assemblies in Scotland, Wales and Northern Ireland exercising certain devolved powers. The UK's total population is 59.6 million, 50 million of whom live in England, 5 million in Scotland, 3 million in Wales, and 1.6 million in Northern Ireland. Nearly one third (18 million) of the UK's total population live in the South-East region of England. Just under 17 million live in the six large English conurbations (Greater London, West Midlands, West Yorkshire, Greater Manchester, Merseyside and Tyne and Wear).

The National Health Service (NHS) was set up in 1948 to provide healthcare for all citizens, based on need, not the ability to pay. It employs 1.35 million staff in Great Britain and is said to be the largest employer in Western Europe. Its annual budget is of the order of £53 billion.

The British Health Service Ombudsman overview and history

Britain's 'Patients' Ombudsman' – formally the Health Service Commissioner – is technically a threesome: there are three Health Service Commissioners, one each for England, Scotland and Wales. Here the offices will be referred to collectively by the generally accepted abbreviation 'HSC'. The HSC was set up in the early 1970s to fill a gap in the then very under-developed complaints arrangements for the NHS. This was achieved by two pieces of legislation: the National Health Service (Scotland) Act 1972 and, for England and Wales, the National Health Service Reorganisation Act 1973.* These measures were subsequently consolidated as

---

* This chapter will deal only with Great Britain. In Northern Ireland the Commissioner for Complaints is also Health Service Commissioner.

the Health Service Commissioners Act 1993. Three years later significant changes to the HSC's jurisdiction were effected by the Health Service Commissioners (Amendment) Act 1996.

The PCA model

As the HSC concept was based on the model of the Parliamentary Ombudsman (formally the Parliamentary Commissioner for Administration – PCA) set up in 1967, we need first to note some key features of the PCA scheme.

The 1967 Ombudsman statute – the Parliamentary Commissioner Act 1967 – had a number of distinctive features. The Ombudsman was styled 'Parliamentary Commissioner for Administration', an officer of Parliament to assist MPs in resolving constituency cases they had been unable to deal with satisfactorily themselves. In consequence, citizens wishing to approach the PCA could only do so through MPs, and his remit was based on matters concerning which MPs could question ministers in Parliament, i.e. ministerial responsibility, and even this was limited in a number of ways. The bodies open to investigation by the PCA were listed in a schedule to the Act, as were a number of matters excluded from his jurisdiction. As an Ombudsman in the classical mode, the PCA was limited to investigating matters of alleged 'maladministration' and inhibited from commenting upon the 'merits' of decisions taken without maladministration. His task was to investigate and report – to the sponsoring MP and Parliament, not the aggrieved citizen.

One of the controversial issues in the debates on the 1967 Act was whether National Health Service hospitals would be included. The Department of Health, reflecting the adamant opposition of the medical profession, was determined that they should not be included. Many MPs, aware from their constituency post-bags of the number of constituents who experienced problems with hospital administrations, were keen that hospitals should be included, not least because the Minister of Health was ministerially responsible for them. In the event, NHS hospitals, like the rest of the National Health Service, were excluded but the decision was a controversial one and led to an immediate inquiry by the newly-established Select Committee on the PCA. However, the Select Committee was not convinced of the necessity for continuing the exclusion and pressure for action on hospital complaints was intensified as a result of a series of Reports of Inquiries into allegations of ill-treatment of patients in psychiatric hospitals, one report specifically recommending the appointment of a Health Service Commissioner.[1,2] The government accordingly included in its NHS reorganisation legislation provisions for establishing Health Service Commissioners for England, for Scotland and for Wales, along the lines of the PCA scheme but with clinical judgement excluded. This legislation was enacted in 1973 and the HSC became operational in October of that year.

Fundamental to the British PCA scheme was, and is, the concept of maladministration, which differentiated 'administrative' complaints from complaints or objections about policy: the PCA would investigate the processes by which decisions were taken, but not their 'merits'. That distinction provided a model for dealing with the problem of 'professional judgement' which exercised the medical professions. If that judgement can be isolated from the processes attendant upon it, then the threat to professional autonomy is much reduced. Following this model, in the HSC legislation the commissioner was excluded from professional judgements but able to investigate complaints of maladministration and service failure by health bodies. Confidence in the viability of this distinction was in part built upon the so-far successful track record of the PCA, who had been at work for five years.

Key differences between the HSC and the PCA

There were, however, some key differences between the PCA and HSC schemes. First, there was no MP filter for the HSC. The only prerequisite was that the health body complained against must have first had an opportunity to comment. MPs who were so protective of their role in relation to complaints against central government departments did not see health service bodies in the same light, notwithstanding the anecdotal evidence from their post-bags of constituents' dissatisfaction with the way in which complaints were being handled. From the start, therefore, complainants have been able to access the Health Service Commissioner direct.

The second key difference from the PCA was that the remit of the HSC was not limited simply to maladministration but extended to service failure: both failure to provide a service and failure in the service provided. At the time of the inception of the HSC scheme, when the scope of the term 'maladministration' was often the subject of criticism, the inclusion of service failure as well as maladministration was seen to be a significant and welcome addition. 'Maladministration' was an unfamiliar term to many and undefined in the statute. It was perceived by some commentators to be obscure and very limited in scope, referring principally if not exclusively to procedural irregularity. Service failure, on the other hand, was a much easier concept for the ordinary citizen to understand, particularly in the context of services to patients for whom inadequate service might cause serious hardship.

In this context it is important to note that the creation of a Health Service Ombudsman in Great Britain did not provide, nor was it intended to provide, patients and users of the NHS services with a 'consumer's advocate' or 'champion'.* In this respect as in others the HSC is a classical Ombudsman: an independent and impartial investigator of complaints whose ability to achieve satisfactory outcomes for complainants depends upon the neutrality which is essential to a thorough, balanced and objective assessment of the evidence. The commissioner may subsequently become an advocate for the remedy that he considers necessary to put right the hardship or injustice which he has found – and in that respect help to remedy the imbalance between the aggrieved complainant and the NHS. But such advocacy is a function of his thorough, balanced and objective investigation and assessment, not of a prior institutional commitment to the interests of the complainant. This subtle but crucial distinction is part of the orthodoxy of classical Ombudsmanship – but it is widely misunderstood by complainants, by patients and consumer organisations, and by NHS professionals and managers.

---

* If anybody has had that role, it was the Community Health Councils and their Scottish equivalents, which were somewhat controversially abolished by the Health and Social Care Act 2001 and replaced by the Patient Advocacy and Liaison Service (PALS).

Evolution of the NHS complaints system

The HSC was, and is, only one part of the NHS procedures for handling complaints. Those procedures, which for historical reasons separated primary care from hospital services, evolved incrementally, not to say haphazardly. Thus, in the primary care sector, in which most practitioners were independent contractors, there was an 'informal' procedure managed by the health authority complementing the formal 'service committee' processes which focused upon whether the terms of the practitioner's contract had been broken. In the hospital sector there was one set of procedures for non-clinical complaints and another for clinical complaints, the latter formalised into a process of 'independent professional review' in 1981. There were also the disciplinary procedures operated by the professions – the General Medical Council (GMC), General Dental Council and so on – which were intended to protect patients against professional misconduct rather than provide specific redress or explanation. And, finally, there was the possibility of litigation, particularly in cases of alleged negligence. The HSC as originally established performed a complementary role in reviewing the handling of complaints about managerial and administrative matters in the hospital sector, but was excluded from dealing with clinical complaints and from those involving family health practitioners.[3]

The Major government's *Citizen's Charter* initiative with its new emphasis upon effective complaint-handling in the public sector led to the commissioning by the government of a comprehensive review of the NHS complaints procedures in 1993. The review report recommended a major restructuring of those procedures, including significant extensions to the Ombudsman's jurisdiction, so as to create a clear and integrated NHS complaints system.[3] The necessary legislation (the Health Service Commissioners [Amendment] Act) was passed in 1996 and currently provides the framework for the Ombudsman's remit.

Although the 1973 legislation provided for separate offices for the PCA and the three HSCs, in practice all four offices have from the outset, and still are, held by the same person and are subject to scrutiny by the same Parliamentary Select Committee. The case for separating the PCA and the HSC as their jurisdictions and caseloads have grown has been reviewed on a number of occasions, including specifically during the revision of the legislative framework in 1996. The government then decided to continue with a joint appointment. However, the issue has arisen again in another form with the proposal, originating from a joint submission by the Parliamentary and English Local Government Ombudsmen, that all the public-sector Ombudsman offices should be brought within one joint scheme. This proposal was endorsed by a Cabinet Office review in April 2000 and subsequently by the select committee. The government announced its acceptance of the proposal in principle in July 2001 but legislation to give it effect has yet to appear.

It is also necessary to note at this point the consequences of devolution to Scotland and Wales. Under the devolution legislation, responsibility for the Health Service Ombudsman arrangements passed to the Scottish Parliament and the National Assembly for Wales. Initially, the existing arrangements continued with little more than a change of title and separate reporting (which complicates statistical comparisons with earlier years). At the time of writing the Scottish Parliament is in the process of legislating to establish a unified public-sector Ombudsman scheme which will incorporate the Scottish Health Service Ombudsman. The government and the National Assembly for Wales have jointly announced that there is to be a review of arrangements in Wales; but this appears to have made little progress.

For the present, however, the Health Service Ombudsman is formally 'at the apex' of the NHS complaints procedure which came into effect in 1996. That procedure has three stages.

1   Stage one (local resolution): initially, a complaint should be made to the person or organisation that provided the service which is the subject of the complaint – an NHS trust, primary care trust, health authority or primary care practitioner. In England in 2000 there were 126 000 such complaints recorded.
2   Stage two (independent review): if the complainant is not satisfied with the outcome of stage one, (s)he may ask for an independent review. When such a request is made, a convener appointed by the health body concerned decides, in consultation with an independent lay person, whether an independent review panel is appropriate. If it is, a panel is brought together to investigate the complaint and produce a written report. Such panels consist of three members – a lay chairman, the convener, and a third, lay member. There were 3457 requests for an independent review in England in 2000, 637 of which resulted in a panel being set up.
3   Stage three (the Ombudsman): if the complainant remains dissatisfied, either with the convener's decision not to convene a panel or with the outcome of the panel investigation, then (s)he may then refer the matter to the Health Service Ombudsman. The Ombudsman must be satisfied that the earlier stages of the complaints procedure have been 'invoked and exhausted', or that there is good reason for them not to have been. The Ombudsman received 2595 cases in 2000 and produced 204 reports of the results of his investigations, as is explained below.

In the year 2001 the Department of Health began a review of the operation of the NHS complaints procedure as part of the government's plan for a 'patient-centred NHS'. As part of the review the department published a discussion document building on the provisions of the Health and Social Care Act 2001.[4] These provisions, which are now being implemented, include the introduction of a Patient Advocacy and Liaison Service (PALS) by every NHS trust with the remit of providing information and on-the-spot help for complainants. This internal mechanism is to be complemented by the Independent Complaints Advocacy Service (ICAS), which will be locally-based but operate to core standards set for the NHS nationwide. PALS and ICAS will not replace the NHS complaints procedure but assist complainants to use it more effectively. The Health Service Ombudsman's role is unaffected, although the more successful PALS and ICAS are in their roles, the less business will presumably need to proceed to the Ombudsman. As these provisions are only now being introduced, it is too early to make any assessment of how they will work in practice.

The period since 1993 has thus been one of considerable change for NHS complaints procedures in general, and the HSC office in particular. The extension of the HSC's remit in 1996 has transformed the nature of his work, as we shall see below. The current government's declared intention to create a unified public sector Ombudsman raises further important organisational questions. So does the continuing review of NHS complaints procedures of which the HSC remains formally the apex.[5,6] Moreover, the government's 1999 White Paper on the NHS brought major developments in clinical governance: a National Institute for Clinical Excellence (NICE) and a Commission for Health Improvement (CHI), with responsibilities to review the management, provision and quality of healthcare provided by the NHS, and to ensure that local management responsibilities for monitoring quality were carried out effectively.[7] In parallel the government began consultations on proposals for reorganising the regulatory arrangements for nurses, midwives and health visitors. At the same time the role of the GMC and its disciplinary and validation procedures have been under close scrutiny as a result of some serious medical failures. As the commissioner has expressed it, the stage is becoming crowded, with a serious risk of duplication of effort and confusion for members of the public.[8] These are serious challenges to which the HSC office will have to respond if it is to build successfully on the foundations laid in its first twenty-five years.

Organisational structure

In this section we shall consider the staffing, financing and accountability of the HSC's office.

Staffing

As indicated in the previous section, the HSC is three Health Service Commissioners in one. Reflecting the relative size of population of the three countries as well as the linkage with the UK Parliamentary Commissioner, the HSC's main office is in London. There are small, separate offices in Edinburgh and Cardiff, both with eight staff, the latter including, as statute requires, some Welsh-speaking staff. Total staff in post for the HSC reached a peak of just over 90 in 1996–97 as the office was building up for the extended jurisdiction. Over the last fifteen years staffing has increased three-fold, reflecting a rapid growth in caseload in the final period of the 'old' jurisdiction and then the impact of the new jurisdiction.

The office is headed by the commissioner and his Health Service deputy. Working to them are five directors. Four of these are investigation directorates, organised on a regional basis, headed by a director with the support of two investigation managers. This new pattern, introduced in April 1998, replaced a format based on the distinction between 'screening' and 'investigation'. This previous pattern reflected the importance in both the PCA and pre-1996 HSC of testing cases received to determine whether they fell within the office's remit – which most then did not because of the clinical judgement and family practitioner service exclusions. With the change in jurisdiction, that division of activity between screening and investigation was found to be no longer appropriate.[9]

The HSC's fifth directorate is the Professional/Clinical Advice Directorate, headed by a director for clinical advice and including the office's internal professional advisers (IPAs). These include six consultants (a physician, a surgeon, and specialists in anaesthetics, psychiatry, accident and emergency medicine, and obstetrics and gynaecology), two general medical practitioners, a general dental practitioner, and a pharmacist. The nursing team includes a senior general nurse, a midwife, a mental health nurse and a senior clinical nurse in child health.[10] In addition to using its IPAs, the office almost always employs external professional advisers (EPAs) to advise on cases which are investigated. These EPAs play a crucial role in the assessment of clinical complaints and their advice to the HSC is published in his final case reports.

Financing

It is not possible to separate the financing of the HSC from that of the PCA. The total expenditure of the office since its establishment is shown in Table 7.1 – note that in 2000–01 it is for England only; the earlier years include Wales and Scotland. The Ombudsman's salary (the post is currently graded at permanent secretary level) is paid out of the consolidated fund in the same way as that of judges. As regards staff, the Ombudsman may appoint such officers as he may determine with the approval of the Treasury as to numbers and conditions of service. In 1977 and 1986 the whole office (i.e. OPCA and OHSC) was subject to a staffing review by the Civil Service Department/Management and Personnel Office. In the mid-1990s a similar process was deployed in the assessment of the additional staffing which would be required for the office's extended remit post-1996. The office is thus subject to the same budgetary disciplines as the civil service and its estimates are presented to Parliament as a separate vote with the parliamentary group (Class XVIII, Vote 1).

Table 7.1 Office of the Parliamentary and Health Service Commissioners: Staffing and Finance, 1996–2001

Year	Staff complement	Total expenditure (£m)
1996–97	220.5	12.72
1997–98	222.4	13.25
1998–99	206.7	12.69
1999–00	209.7	13.57
2000–01	219.5	12.46

Source OPCA/OHSC Secretariat.

Accountability

In terms of accountability, one would have expected that since the HSC scheme was modelled on that of the PCA, the HSC should therefore be considered accountable to Parliament. However, the issue was not quite as clear-cut as that, since the 1972–73 legislation rather blurred the picture with the provision that the HSC should report to Parliament through the secretary of state (1993 Act, s14[3] and [4]). This was a relic of the Department of Health's initial preference when beginning the drafting of the legislation for a Departmental Commissioner. In practice, the institutional linkage with the PCA determined that the line of accountability would be the same – i.e. to the select committee – and this was given statutory recognition in the 1996 Act.

We can, therefore, now say unambiguously that the HSC reports directly to Parliament. As with the PCA he may from time to time lay occasional and 'special' reports before each House of Parliament, and is required to lay annually a general report on the performance of his functions before both houses. In the narrower sense of having an obligation to respond to complaints and representations about the actions of the office, accountability is in practice exercised through the associated select committee of the House of Commons. Thus on occasion the committee – until recently the Select Committee on the Parliamentary Commissioner for Administration but currently the Select Committee on Public Administration with a rather wider remit – hears and considers expressions of opinion about the performance of the HSC, and expects the HSC in turn to respond to its conclusions and recommendations. In most parliamentary sessions the select committee holds a hearing on the HSC's annual report at which he is invited to draw the committee's attention to any matters of particular significance. This helps the committee to schedule its programme of work, which will often include following with particular health authorities and the NHS management executive matters raised by the commissioner – both particular cases and more general quality of service issues.

As indicated earlier the select committee can take some credit for the part it played in the setting up of the HSC scheme following the exclusion of the NHS from the PCA's remit. Since then the committee has been persistent in its support of pressure to widen the HSC's jurisdiction. Its review of the PCA and HSC in 1993 argued that the HSC should be seen as the apex of a unified NHS complaints system and that his remit should encompass family practitioner services as well as the operation of the formal complaints procedures of Family Health Service Authorities.[11] These recommendations were explicitly endorsed by the Wilson Committee, subsequently adopted by the government, and enacted in the Health Service Commissioners (Amendment) Act 1996.[12,13]

As with the PCA, the select committee plays an important role in backing up the HSC's findings and recommendations in those cases where health service authorities are reluctant to accept them and in following through on action taken to ensure that the appropriate lessons are learned from these cases of maladministration or service failure.

The Ombudsman, it should be noted, is also subject to judicial review by the courts. In view of the wide discretionary powers conferred on the office, however, the courts have been very reluctant to find for complainants seeking to challenge the Ombudsman's decisions (for example, as regards jurisdictional issues) and, one case apart, are generally unlikely to be successful.[14] In a recent challenge to the HSC's powers to summon a clinical practitioner to give evidence in connection with a complaint, on the grounds that the commissioner did not have the power to investigate the case and that the matters concerned would involve a breach of confidentiality, the court held firmly and decisively in the commissioner's favour.[15]

Role and function

In this section we shall consider first jurisdiction, second powers of investigation, third competence and, finally, improving the quality of administration.

Jurisdiction

As mentioned above, the HSC scheme has been subject to major changes as a result of the enactment of the Health Service Commissioners (Amendment) Act 1996. These changes involved major extensions to the HSC's jurisdiction which have only recently fed through into the commissioner's caseload. In addition, the HSC accepted a role under the government's access to official information (AOI) policy. This account of the HSC scheme's role and function is in three parts: the first deals with the provisions prior to 1996; the second with AOI; and the third part then sets out the position brought about by the 1996 legislation.

The pre-1996 framework

The HSC's general remit was defined in section 3 of the 1993 Act in terms of the type of complaints he was empowered to investigate. To qualify, a complaint had to be made by or on behalf of a person that he had sustained injustice or hardship in consequence of:

- a failure in a service provided by a health service body
- a failure of such a body to provide a service which it was the function of the body to provide
- maladministration connected with any other action taken by or on behalf of such a body.

As with the PCA, the HSC was not empowered to question the merits of a decision taken without maladministration.

In the original legislation four categories of matters were excluded from investigation by the HSC. Two of these excluded categories, matters of clinical judgement and actions by family service practitioners (general practitioners, dentists, opticians and pharmacists), were brought within the HSC's remit by the 1996 Act. The other two were, first, matters where an alternative remedy is available, namely [1993 Act, s4]:

- matters in relation to which the aggrieved person has or had a right of appeal, reference or review to a tribunal, a remedy by proceedings in a court of law – unless the HSC is satisfied that in the particular circumstances it is not reasonable to expect that the aggrieved person should use these alternatives
- action which is the subject of a special statutory inquiry initiated by the secretary of state
- action which is covered by the protective functions of the Mental Welfare Commission for Scotland.

The remaining category excludes personnel and contractual matters, with two important exceptions [1993 Act, s7]:

- NHS contracts for community care
- matters arising from arrangements by NHS bodies with a non-NHS body to provide services for patients.

In addition to those jurisdictional tests, for a complaint to be investigable by the HSC, the 1993 Act [s9] laid down four procedural requirements. Complaints must be made in writing by either the aggrieved person or, where that person had died or was for any reason unable to act for himself, by his personal representative, a member of his family, or some body or individual suitable to represent him. They must be made within a year of the date on which the aggrieved person was first aware of the matters alleged, but the HSC was given discretion to accept complaints made after this deadline where he judged it reasonable to do so. Fourthly, before he could proceed to investigate a complaint the HSC was required by the original legislation to satisfy himself that it had been brought to the notice of the health service body concerned and that that body had been afforded a reasonable opportunity to investigate it. (Different provisions were introduced by the 1996 Act.)

Access to official information

The introduction of codes of access to official information was part of the Major government's *Citizen's Charter*. The 1993 White Paper *Open Government* [Cm 2290] declared the government's intention to achieve greater public access to official information through non-statutory codes rather than a Freedom of Information Act as advocated by freedom of information campaigners. The White Paper included a commitment that the NHS should have its own code and an NHS *Code of Practice on Openness in the NHS in England* was published in April 1995. Similar codes were introduced in Scotland and Wales.

Before the codes came into effect, at the request of the then Health Secretary Virginia Bottomley, in 1995 the then HSC Sir William Reid agreed to undertake responsibility for investigating complaints from members of the public that their requests for information under the NHS codes had not been met. As PCA he had already taken on a similar responsibility in relation to the government's *Code of Practice on Access to Government Information*. In order to publicise his new responsibilities in July 1995 Sir William issued a revised version of the leaflet *How the Health Service Ombudsman Can Help You,* setting out his powers and explaining that he could now investigate complaints of non-disclosure under the codes. He and his staff also made references to this extension of HSC jurisdiction in articles and speeches. Sir William also wrote to the chief executives of health authorities, boards and trusts in England, Scotland and Wales, and to other health bodies in his remit, in order to explain how he intended to handle complaints about non-disclosure. When in April 1996 the HSC's jurisdiction was extended to include NHS family health service practitioners, Sir William also included information about his responsibilities for investigating complaints under the codes when writing to explain to them how the new legislation had brought their activities within his remit.

In his 1995–96 annual report Sir William drew attention to the key features of his new jurisdiction. First, the codes were non-statutory. The HSC's powers to investigate complaints under them therefore lay in his general remit to investigate maladministration and service failure under the Health Service Commissioner Acts. Failure by an NHS body to release information under the NHS code of openness was maladministration unless covered by the exemptions allowed under the code. One important difference from the HSC's general remit, however, was that in other complaints complainants were expected to show some *prima facie* reason to have suffered some hardship or injustice. But in relation to complaints about non-disclosure under the codes Sir William regarded a refusal to provide information to which the complainant believed that there was an entitlement under the codes as of itself grounds on which to claim injustice or hardship. This approach mirrored his practice as PCA in relation to the *Code of Practice on Access to Government Information.*[16]

Sir William also drew attention to the fact that the NHS codes, like the government code, were expressed in terms of information, not documents. The underlying principle of the codes was that information would be made available unless it could be shown to fall within one or more of the nine exemptions set out in the codes. In respect of some of those exemptions health bodies were expected to consider whether there was a public interest case for disclosing information which would otherwise be exempt.[17]

To date the HSC has received very few complaints or enquiries about access to information. In November 1996 he reported to Parliament that in the first sixteen months of his new remit he had received only 31 written representations. Of these 10 were enquiries. Of the 21 complaints, he had investigated three and begun an investigation into a fourth, which he had discontinued when the complainant decided to take legal action against the health body concerned.[18] The HSC commented that this number of complaints was even lower than the number made to him about access to government information. In the HSC's opinion these low numbers were the result of a mixture of apathy, the hurdles complainants have to surmount before they can come to him, and the lack of any sustained publicity for the codes from government and the NHS.[19] The position has not changed in subsequent years. When the current government's Freedom of Information Act comes fully into effect, these responsibilities will transfer to the new information commissioner.

The 1996 amendments
The 1996 Act fundamentally changed the Health Service Commissioner's office. It made three main jurisdictional changes and widened the role and function of the office very substantially. The first change extended the HSC's jurisdiction to include family health service providers (i.e. family doctors, general dental practitioners, opticians and pharmacists), the Mental Health Welfare Commission for Scotland (which oversees the welfare of detained patients), and independent health service providers (where these are treating NHS patients).

The second change removed the exclusion of matters of clinical judgement from the HSC's remit. The HSC is now permitted to investigate matters of clinical judgement, including the merits of clinical decisions, though he remains debarred from investigating the merits of administrative decisions. This was the area which was most fiercely contested by the medical profession. It was also the area which prior to the new statute yielded the highest number of rejections by the HSC of cases as outwith his statutory jurisdiction.

The third change made in 1996 followed from the government's decision to accept the Wilson Committee's recommendation to establish a two-stage complaints procedure within the NHS, which would be overseen by the HSC.[20] Under the 1996 Act complainants still have direct access to the HSC but he cannot accept cases for investigation until he is satisfied that the earlier stages of the complaints procedures have been 'invoked and exhausted', unless he believes that in the particular circumstances it would not be reasonable to expect the complainant to have done so. Thus he has discretion to decide in a particular case to override the general requirement that local complaints procedures should be exhausted.

The 1996 changes have taken the HSC into three new areas: clinical judgement, general practice, and oversight of the NHS complaints system as a whole. Cases arising in these areas began to be reported upon in 1998 and now form the over-whelming majority of the caseload. Of the 204 investigation reports completed in 2000–01, 77% concerned matters of clinical judgement.[21]

Powers of investigation

The 1996 Act places the HSC at the apex of a more integrated NHS complaints system. Not only does this give an avenue of appeal to the complainant who is dis-satisfied with the outcome of the first two stages of the system, it could also give to the HSC an important role in setting and monitoring standards for complaint-handling across the NHS as a whole – if the cases reaching him are in any way typical.

The HSC's powers of investigation follow closely those granted to the PCA. A commissioner may certify an offence to the court where a person without lawful excuse obstructs him or any of his officers in the performance of his functions or is guilty of any act or omission in relation to an investigation which, if that were a proceeding in court, would constitute a contempt. Where an offence is so certified, the court may inquire into the matter and, after hearing any relevant witnesses and any statement that may be offered in defence, deal with the offence as if it had been a contempt of court (1993 Act, s13).

Where the HSC proposes to conduct an investigation into a complaint, he must afford to the health service body concerned, and to any other person who is alleged in the complaint to have taken or authorised the action complained of, an opportunity to comment on any allegations contained in the complaint (1993 Act, s11[1]). The 'invoked and exhausted' provision in the 1996 Act makes this much more straightforward in most cases.

Every investigation must be conducted in private but in other respects the procedure shall be such as the HSC considers appropriate in the circumstances of the case. In particular, he may obtain information from such persons and in such manner, and may make such enquiries, as he thinks fit, and he may determine whether any person may be legally represented (1993 Act, s11[2] and [3]).

For the purposes of an investigation an HSC may require any officer or member of the health service body concerned, or any other person who in his opinion is able to supply information or produce documents relevant to the investigation, to supply any such information or produce any such document. The HSC has the same powers as the court in respect of the attendance and examination of witnesses (including the administration of oaths and affirmations and the examination of witnesses abroad) and the production of documents (1993 Act, s12[1] and [2]).

These powers override the obligations, whether statutory or otherwise, on crown servants to maintain secrecy or confidentiality, and the crown is not entitled to make claims of privilege in relation to the production of documents or the giving of evidence (1993 Act, s12[3] and [4]). However, as with the PCA, cabinet and cabinet committee proceedings and documents are beyond the HSC's reach (1993 Act, s12[5]) – though for the HSC this point is largely academic.

The totality of these powers gives the HSC virtually unrestricted access to papers and persons. What it does not do is ensure that the relevant health service bodies can supply those papers or persons. A recurrent theme in HSC reports concerns the unavailability of records or the inability to track down particular personnel who are no longer in the employ of the health service body concerned.

Competence

An important issue in the analysis of Ombudsman schemes is the basis upon which the Ombudsman can make criticisms of, and in consequence propose remedies for, the actions of public authorities. The HSC has three quarries in which he may seek grounds for criticism of the actions of the bodies he investigates. These grounds are set out in section 3(1) of the 1993 Act. In addition to maladministration, the HSC is also empowered to investigate complaints that a person has sustained injustice or hardship in consequence of a failure in service provided by a health service body or a failure to provide a service which it is the function of that body to provide.

The inclusion of service failure significantly widened the HSC's remit in comparison with the PCA. The growing use of published service standards, first introduced under the *Patient's Charter* initiative, has made the qualitative aspect of judgement more straightforward, though on occasions it has proved complex when service provision is (said to be) affected by resource constraints. A recent comment by the HSC on his approach to the exercise of clinical judgement illustrates the realism which successive HSCs have had to bring to the issue of the impact of resource constraints on allegations of service failure. The commissioner stated, 'I do not view complaints from an ivory tower oblivious of shortages of resources and the stress under which many hospital staff work … (my concern is) to establish whether what happened was within the bounds of reasonable care in the circumstances prevailing at the time'.[22] Thus in one case although he considered the delay in providing anaesthetist attention to a patient unacceptable, he did not criticise the staff involved for giving priority to other patients with still more urgent needs.[23]

Improving the quality of administration

A frequently cited role of Ombudsman schemes is, through the investigation and remedying of administrative faults, to help to bring about an improvement in the quality of administration. This is often closely linked with the Ombudsman's perceived ability to be able to identify and propose remedies for systemic faults in administrative and service delivery processes. In Great Britain it has certainly been true that some holders of the office of HSC have seen this as a significant part of their role. Sir William Reid, for example, had a particular concern with the wider administrative implications of the results of his investigations. His special report on Salford was issued specifically so that 'all NHS bodies will draw useful lessons about handling complaints from this report'.[24] A key feature of the HSC's work in this regard is the publication at six-monthly intervals of a selection of reports on completed investigations. In his preface to one such selection, the HSC stated: 'In publishing a selection of my reports on completed investigations I bring the results of my enquiries to a wider audience who can benefit from the experience of others. Some good thereby comes from events which have caused distress'.[25]

The extent of the impact of the HSC's activities under this heading is hard to judge. It is clear that the select committee has an important role to play in reinforcing the HSC's findings and bringing greater public (i.e. media) attention to them. This is evident in the way in which the Salford cases were dealt with and it is a feature of the committee's hearings on the HSC's annual reports that health authorities, both locally and nationally, are called upon to explain their failures and, more particularly, whether appropriate actions have been taken to prevent recurrences.

As explained above the 1996 Act placed the HSC at the apex of a more integrated NHS complaints system and gave him the opportunity for an important role in setting and monitoring standards for complaint-handling across the NHS as a whole. Failures in this area were a fertile ground for complaints to the HSC long before the 1996 changes. The advent of the *Patient's Charter* brought awareness not only of the right to complain but also of the difficulties complainants continued to find in exercising that right. Implementing the new procedures has shown how much still needs to be done to ensure that service providers, managers and senior administrators take seriously their responsibilities for effective complaint-handling. It is not sufficient to draw up procedures. They have also to be effectively implemented, which includes an appropriate level of monitoring by senior managers.

There is, however, a very significant limitation to the role that the HSC can play in regard to improving the quality of service provided by the NHS: the tiny volume of cases that it sees cannot be considered in any way typical. This was always the case and it is even more so with the 'invoked and exhausted' requirement of the 1996 Act. What the HSC sees are the exceptions. His investigations may reveal systemic problems at a particular time in a particular hospital, health authority, GP or dental practice but who can know whether these are typical? From the investigations it conducts, the office will undoubtedly gain useful insights into the workings or non-workings of NHS procedures. But these insights have to be fed into the wider framework of quality management in the NHS in order to be evaluated. In this respect the current exploration of service standards – and particularly one relating to complaint-handling itself – may prove particularly illuminating on the likely effectiveness of the HSC's role in this area.

The work of the HSC

A feature of the work of the HSC has been the variability of its workload. In the mid-1980s during Sir Anthony Barrowclough's term of office, there was a sharp (14%) increase in the number of complaints in his first year followed by a decline in each successive year to reach a low of 753 – i.e. 8% fewer than in his first year in office. At the same time the average number of grievances per results report issued increased from 3.5 to 4 and the uphold rate increased from 47% to 61%. Thus during the 1980s as a whole the volume of cases received rose by 16% (from 647 to 753), grievances investigated by 39% (from 399 to 556) and results reports issued by 23% (from 113 to 139). This marked increase in output continued under Sir William Reid with a rise to an all-time high of 229 reports in 1995–96 – a growth of 65%. Over the same period, the number of cases received increased by 80% (from 990 to 1784) and the number of grievances investigated increased by 12% (from 487 to 546), reflecting Sir William's declared policy of more focused investigations. During his period in office the uphold rate also increased significantly, from 48.5% to 62%.

The second half of the 1990s have seen the consequences of the changes to the HSC's jurisdiction working through – which, incidentally, means that extreme care has to be exercised when making comparisons between pre- and post-1996 figures. Cases received, which had been rising strongly throughout the 1990s, continued their steep upward climb, rising by 61% in 1998–99 to reach 2869, compared with 1784 in 1995–96. But as the effects of new jurisdiction worked their way through, cases received fell back to 2536 in 1999–2000, increasing slightly to 2595 in 2000–01. More significantly, the proportion of cases accepted for investigation was falling significantly at the end of Sir William Reid's period of office: 11% in 1995–96 became 6% the following year and 4% in 1997–98.[26] Since then there has been a noticeable increase – to 9% in 2000–01 – which reflects a deliberate change of policy by the commissioner to widen the criteria for acceptability.[27,28] Similarly, results reports issued, which had increased to 238 in 1996–97, fell to 119 (98 for England only) in 1998–99 but recovered to 147 (128 for England only) the following year and 204 for England only in 2000–01.

As mentioned earlier, since the coming into effect of the 1996 Act the make-up of the caseload has changed very significantly, with clinical complaints now accounting for more than three-quarters of the caseload. We can assess the picture prior to that time by looking at the analysis of subjects and service areas of grievances investigated in 1995–96, which showed a predominance of grievances concerning hospital acute inpatient services (60%), as regards service area, and that hospital complaint-handling was the leading topic (27%) closely followed by care and treatment (24%). The difference made by the inclusion of general medical and dental services can be seen from Table 7.2.

Table 7.2 Total number of grievances in investigations completed by Health Service Ombudsman in England by service area*

Service area	1995–96	2000–01
Hospital inpatient	271	128
Hospital outpatient	59	29
Hospital A & E	24	7
Geriatric	12	0
Mental health	25	20
Maternity	14	3
Ambulance	18	11
General medical services	0**	83
General dental services	0**	16
Other community health	3	14
Administrative/Other	120	32
Total	546	343

* 1995–96 was the year before the Ombudsman's jurisdiction was widened to include matters of clinical judgement and complaints against family service practitioners.
** Not within jurisdiction.
Source HSC Annual Reports.

Little is available by way of a socio-economic analysis of the background of complainants but the office does produce an annual analysis of their geographical origin. There seems to be a marked disparity, with the highest number of complaints coming from London and the South-East; in 2000–01 more than 42% of English complaints came from these two regions, but since these account for some 36% of the population the disparity is, perhaps, more apparent than real.[29]

Compliance and remedies

Turning to compliance and remedies, the office appears to have an impressive record, though it is difficult to obtain verifiable information on complainants' satisfaction. In terms of remedies, like any classical Ombudsman the HSC is empowered (only) to investigate and to report. The 1993 Act provides (s14[1]) that the HSC shall send a report of the results of an investigation by him to:

- the person who made the complaint
- any MP who to the HSC's knowledge assisted in the making of the complaint (or if he is no longer an MP to such other MP as the HSC thinks appropriate)
- the health service body concerned
- any person who is alleged in the complaint to have taken or authorised the action complained of
- if the body concerned is not a district health authority, the Secretary of State.

If the HSC decides not to conduct an investigation, he is required (1993 Act, s14[2]) to send a statement of his reasons to the complainant and to any MP who assisted in the making of the complaint. Until the passage of the 1996 Act the HSC was also required to send a statement to the health service body concerned. If after conducting an investigation it appears to the HSC that the injustice or hardship sustained by the person aggrieved has not been and will not be remedied, he is empowered (1993 Act, s14[3]) to make a special report. In the original legislation such a report was made to the secretary of state who was required 'as soon as is reasonably practical' to lay a copy of the report before each House of Parliament. The 1996 Act removed the secretary of state from this process so that the HSC himself now lays any special report he may make before each House of Parliament.

Prior to the 1996 changes, in 2485 results reports issued the HSC has upheld more than half the grievances investigated – 4365 (51.7%) out of 8443. In the vast majority of cases the remedy achieved for the complainant – apart from the vindication of the grievance being upheld – was an apology from the health service body concerned. To illustrate this from the periods of office of successive HSCs, an apology was the remedy accepted by Cecil Clothier in 90 out of 110 cases in 1983–84; in 109 out of 123 cases by Sir Anthony Barrowclough in 1988–89; and in 72 cases by William Reid in 1989–90.[30–32]

Not all complainants find this procedure satisfactory. Some object in particular to the fact that the apology is conveyed to them by the HSC rather than made by the health service body itself. One dissatisfied complainant in 1984 pursued this aspect not only with the HSC and his office but also his MP and the chairman of the select committee. The HSC argued that routing the apology through his office ensured that it was in the appropriate terms and not 'modified or expressed in so perfunctory a way as to leave the complainant wondering whether an apology has in fact been given'.[33] But some complainants wonder how they could be sure that the authority concerned really did 'regret' what had occurred if the authority itself had not expressed the regret.

In a small minority of cases the HSC concluded that reimbursement for financial loss would be a proper response and invited the health authority to make an ex-gratia payment. The sums involved have not been large – they range from £25 to £20 000.[34] It is important to distinguish such payments from compensation for a legal wrong: if that is what a complainant is seeking, then it is unlikely that the HSC would take the case since 'such a remedy – usually linked to an accusation of negligence – is for the courts, not me, to decide'.[35] This is, of course, a particularly significant aspect with complaints about clinical judgement.

Again following the classical Ombudsman model, the HSC has no statutory powers relating to enforcement. His only 'disciplinary sanction' lies in the making of reports, which are of two kinds. Most reports (i.e. not 'special reports' as defined by the Act) go to the next higher level of the NHS or the secretary of state himself (and in recent years the NHS chief executive); this is itself a significant bureaucratic sanction. It does encourage health service managers to accept the HSC's findings, which is what happens in the vast majority of cases.

In the very few cases where the HSC has been unable to persuade the health authority to provide the remedy he has recommended, the cases will be brought to the select committee. Such cases are exceptional. The overwhelming picture is one of willingness on the part of health authority managers and professionals to accept the HSC's findings and comply with his recommendations. And the presence of the select committee in the background usually brings even the tiny reluctant minority into line. When dealing with administrative errors by government departments or other public authorities, support from Parliament, and in particular the commons select committee, gives the HSC, like the PCA, significant additional leverage to persuade reluctant chief executives and senior managers of the practical wisdom of accepting critical reports and going along with the commissioner's recommendations.

However, clinical judgement is a different matter, one in which the procedures of political and administrative accountability may not seem so apposite, particularly to hospital clinicians and family practitioners. In some cases, such as two cited in his November 1998 report, the GP concerned did not agree with the HSC's findings and declined to apologise for all the matters he criticised.[36] For the aggrieved complainant an Ombudsman report finding in his favour is hardly a remedy if the practitioner concerned declines even to apologise. Is the (justified) complainant to be left without a mechanism to achieve compliance in such cases? Perhaps not: the HSC has himself pointed to one possibility. Although in such cases he has so far only identified the health authority area in which the GP worked, and not actually named the individual GP or dentist, he does reserve the right to name individuals in future if circumstances warrant it.[37] The 'mobilisation of shame', as the Netherlands Ombudsman Marten Oosting has observed, is a key element in an Ombudsman's armoury. How it is deployed will be a key factor in the development of this new aspect of the HSC's jurisdiction. As it happened one of the cases reported in November 1998 led to the GP concerned being called before the select committee. The GP was criticised by the commissioner for failing to visit a patient in response to a call to his emergency answering service and for his standard of record-keeping, for which he apologised and agreed to take appropriate remedial action.[38] This was the committee's first opportunity to review a case in which the commissioner had investigated a doctor's clinical judgement.[39] Press reports of the hearing named the doctor but the committee – in its subsequent report on the PCA's annual report, but referring specifically to the GP's case – was keen to disavow a 'naming and shaming' approach: 'It is not and has not been the Committee's intention to "name and shame". It is the salutary lessons to be drawn from individual cases that we are interested in.'[40] Nevertheless, such reporting (the GP's name and area were printed in the select committee's report) will be a powerful inducement to any practitioners criticised by the Ombudsman to agree to the remedy he proposes in the hope of avoiding the risk of adverse publicity arising from such a select committee hearing.

It was a different story, however, in the case of a dental practitioner case reported in November 1999. The commissioner, drawing on the reports of his assessors, found that Mr Capon's record-keeping lacked thoroughness and that he had not adequately assessed and treated the complainant's tooth decay and gum disease. However, Mr Capon did not accept the commissioner's invitation to apologise to the complainant nor did he agree to act on the recommendation that he consider ways to improve his understanding of current practice in the treatment of periodontal disease.[41] This refusal to accept the commissioner's findings was the subject of adverse comment from the select committee in December 2000, which was endorsed in the response from the secretary of state's reply to the committee the following March.[42,43]

The HSC is also empowered to lay 'special reports' before Parliament (directly since 1996, via the secretary of state before then) if, after his investigation, it appears to him that the person aggrieved has sustained injustice and hardship which will not be remedied. In June 1996 the HSC published two such reports. One was a systemic investigation into complaint-handling by a particular trust which was generating an unusual volume of complaints and whose performance had already been considered by the select committee.[44]

The second special report concerned complaints about arrangements for providing long-term healthcare, which included his findings of five of several complaints he had investigated since an earlier special report in 1994 on a case involving the failure of Leeds Health Authority to provide long-term NHS care for a brain-damaged patient. In his conclusion the HSC commented: 'My aim in publishing these cases, and previous ones, is to illustrate the issues involved and how mistakes can be avoided. I hope that the cases in this volume will demonstrate some of the administrative problems, and the difficulties which can be caused for the individuals concerned'.[45]

Assessment and conclusion

From an institutional point of view the British Health Service Ombudsman offices face an uncertain future. Devolution, recent developments in the NHS and governance, the emergence of PALS, ICAS and bodies like CHI and the government's endorsement of the concept of a unified public-sector Ombudsman scheme raise the question of what the distinctive contribution of a 'Health Service Ombudsman office' should now be. The present commissioner is clear that the 'core role' is to deal with complaints and it is therefore in that context that the office should currently be assessed.[46]

In its British form the Health Service Ombudsman is a classical Ombudsman, not a mediator or patient advocate. The HSC stands at the apex of a quite complex complaints system, the earlier stages of which handle the overwhelming majority (*ca*. 98%) of patients' complaints. In that context the strengths of the British HSC scheme are:

- the impartiality and independence of the Ombudsman
- the virtually unrestricted powers of investigation, resulting in thorough and authoritative reports
- the flexibility with which the terms 'maladministration' and 'service failure' have been interpreted, with the result that the HSC has been able to criticise a wide range of administrative and managerial actions
- the effectiveness of the HSC in securing compliance with his recommendations for redress for individual complainants and for improvements in administrative systems and practices
- the supportive relationship with the select committee which underpins the continuing effectiveness of the scheme.

The changes made in 1996 removed what until then had been the HSC's major weakness – limited jurisdiction. Given that, the two features now most open to criticism would appear to be its visibility and inaccessibility for the majority of complainants and the time which the office takes to complete investigations and issue reports. Thus the HSC faces the two challenges which confront most Ombudsman offices: making itself accessible and producing reports quickly enough to satisfy complainants but not so fast as to sacrifice the thoroughness without which their credibility with the body complained against would be undermined. Neither of these issues is straightforward. How does one measure the extent of visibility and accessibility? The conventional way – recognition polls – begs the question at what point is it necessary or appropriate for a patient or relative to consider themselves a potential complainant needing to know how and to whom to address a complaint should something go wrong.

A great deal of effort has been invested by the HSC and the NHS in recent years in making available leaflets and similar literature so that potential complainants can easily discover what they need to know. But the commissioner's own investigations have shown that implementation of the NHS complaints procedures has been far from complete or universal. In that situation the role of intermediate bodies such as citizens advice bureaux and community health councils (CHCs) is crucial. How the replacement of CHCs by 'PALS' and the work of ICAS will affect the position will be an important question in the next few years.

The task of informing the public at large how to access the HSC is a ceaseless but necessary enterprise, common to all Ombudsman systems. A Central Office of Information research report on general public awareness of the office in 1996 found that only 9% made an unprompted mention of the Ombudsman when asked who they could think of who could look at their complaint against the NHS, and that awareness was higher among men, those aged over 35 and in social grades A and B. Claimed awareness rose to 48% when mention was made of the Health Service Ombudsman. But general awareness is not necessarily the best indicator. What matters is the visibility and accessibility of a complaints mechanism at the point at which a service user has a problem s/he wants to complain about. And there is a particular need to reach out to the vulnerable and disadvantaged sections of the community. This is doubly important in the health sector as these sections of the community frequently have special health needs. Vulnerability in this context has many forms: physical and mental handicap, the frailty of the very old and the very young, non-native English speakers, the educationally disadvantaged. To such people negotiating bureaucratic systems is always a challenge. When things go wrong for them, it is essential that they, or those who represent or assist them, have easy access to complaints procedures.

'When things go wrong': the need to focus on that point in time is especially relevant to the Health Service Ombudsman which (normally) comes into play only when the internal NHS procedures have been 'invoked and exhausted'. That provision makes the NHS itself the gateway to the Ombudsman. If in 2001 one asks patients and consumer organisations about the accessibility of the Health Service Ombudsman, they are likely (in the opinion of the current Deputy Health Service Ombudsman) to reply that in practice it is of no great moment. What matters is accessibility to the NHS complaints procedure. There are tens of millions of contacts with the NHS every year, but only about 135 000 complaints. The major reason why there are not more is that people are too frightened to complain.[47] On that analysis, the appropriate route to raising the profile of the Ombudsman's office would seem to lie in focusing attention upon two groups of people: first, patient representative organisations and citizens' advocacy groups (hence PALS and ICAS) and, second, NHS practitioners, because they also often act as advocates for their patients.

Another key factor affecting potential complainants' decisions whether to access a complaints procedure is the 'hassle factor': how much time and effort will be involved and is it likely to be productive? In that calculation, the amount of time that is likely to elapse before the outcome is known will be an important factor. Complainants are likely to be put off by the prospect of their case 'dragging on and on', particularly if the content or context of their complaint is itself emotionally distressing, which is often so in the health field. And since complainants will normally have been through the first two stages of the NHS complaints procedure before approaching the HSC, there has already been a significant lapse of time.

Under constant pressure from the select committee, patient and consumer organisations, successive commissioners have tried to reduce throughput times, with mixed results. The concentrated efforts to deal with backlogs in the mid-1990s seemed to be successful, but the changed jurisdiction has made subsequent comparisons invalid. The current commissioner has been rightly cautious about promising more rapid progress. But the fact remains that a complainant taking his case to the HSC is likely to have to wait many months before the commissioner's report on that case is available, and those many months will be in addition to the time already taken exhausting the NHS complaints procedure.

At the start of the twenty-first century the Office of the Health Service Ombudsman, to use its preferred but still unofficial title, faces significant challenges if it is to build successfully upon the substantial foundations laid in the period prior to the 1996 Act. The office has a substantial legacy but it has some stiff challenges to face if it is to continue to provide an effective complaint-handling service for health service users. Whether that service is provided as an independent office or, as seems likely, as part of a team of public sector Ombudsmen, it must be a service which is easy to access and produces timely and fair results for both complainants and those complained against. Justice demands no less.

References

1 *Second Report of the Select Committee on the PCA* (1968) HC 350, 1967–68. HMSO, London, paras 36–37.
2 *Report of the Committee of Inquiry into Farleigh Hospital* (1971) Cmnd 4557. HMSO, London, p. 29.
3 Department of Health (1994) *Wilson Report. Being Heard*. HMSO, London.
4 Department of Health (2001) *Involving Patients and the Public in Healthcare: a discussion document*. HMSO, London.
5 Department of Health (2001) *The NHS Complaints Procedure National Evaluation*. HMSO, London.
6 Department of Health (2001) *Reforming the NHS Complaints Procedure: a listening document*. HMSO, London.
7 Department of Health (1999) *The New NHS: modern, dependable*. Cm 3807. The Stationery Office, London.
8 *Annual Report 1998–99*, HSC, p. 26.
9 *Annual Report 1997–98*, HSC, para. 1.11.
10 *Annual Report 2000–01*, HSC, Annex B.
11 First Report of the Select Committee (1994) *The Powers, Work and Jurisdiction of the Ombudsman*. HC 33, 1993–94. HMSO, London.
12 Op. cit., p. 67.
13 Department of Health (1995) *Acting on Complaints*. HMSO, London, pp. 6–7.
14 Giddings P (2000) Ex p. Balchin: findings of maladministration and injustice. *Public Law*: 201–4.
15 *Hession v Health Service Commissioner for Wales*, May 2001.
16 *Annual Report 1995–96*, HSC, para. 5.6.
17 Ibid., para. 5.9.
18 Health Service Commissioner (1997) *Selected Investigations: access to official information in the National Health Service*. HC 62, 1996–97. HMSO, London, para. 14.
19 Ibid., para. 18.
20 Department of Health (1995) *Acting on Complaints*. HMSO, London, p. 3.
21 *Annual Report 2000–01*, HSC, p. 1. (This refers to England only.)
22 Health Service Commissioner (1998) *Investigations Completed April–September 1998*. HC 3, 1998–99. HMSO, London, pp. 5–6.
23 Ibid., p. 6.
24 Health Service Commissioner (1996) *Second Report, 1995–96. Investigation of Complaint-handling by Salford Royal Hospitals NHS Trust*. HC 429. HMSO, London, para. 5.
25 Health Service Commissioner (1996) *Third Report, 1995–96: Selected Investigations Completed October 1995 to March 1996*. HC 464. HMSO, London, p. iii.
26 *Annual Report 1999–2000*, HSC, p. 37.
27 Ibid., para. 5.7.
28 *Annual Report 2000–01*, HSC, p. 1.
29 *Annual Report 2000–01*, HSC, p. 20.
30 *Annual Report 1983–84*, HSC, para. 129.
31 *Annual Report 1988–89*, HSC, para. 99.
32 *Annual Report 1989-90*, HSC, para. 67.
33 *Annual Report 1983–84*, HSC, para. 129.

34 *Annual Report 1989–90*, HSC.

35 Ibid., para. 68.

36 Health Service Commissioner (1998) *Investigations Completed April–September 1998*. HC 3, 1998–99. HMSO, London, Cases S 42/97–98 and E 1934/97–98.

37 Ibid., p. 6.

38 Case E 1253/96–97.

39 Select Committee (1999) *Second Report for 1998–99*, paras 41–42, and *Evidence*, pp. 103–13.

40 Select Committee (1999) HC 136, 1998–99, para. 34.

41 Case E 544/98–99 reported in HSC (1999) *Investigations Completed, April–September 1999*. HC 19, 1999–2000, pp. 74–9.

42 Select Committee (2000) *First Report for 2000–2001*, para. 8.

43 Select Committee (2001) *Second Special Report 2000–2001, Memorandum from the Secretary of State for Health*, p. 1.

44 Health Service Commissioner (1996) *Second Report, 1995–96. Investigation of Complaint-handling by Salford Royal Hospitals NHS Trust*. HC 429. HMSO, London.

45 Health Service Commissioner (1996) *Fifth Report, 1995–96. Investigations of Complaints about Long Term NHS Care*. HC 504. HMSO, London, para. 9.

46 *Annual Report 1998–99*, HSC, p. 26.

47 Hilary Scott, interview, 24 August 2001.

CHAPTER 8

Conclusion

Lars Fallberg and Stephen Mackenney

The Patient Ombudsman as an instrument for implementing patients' rights

The weak point of any law protecting the rights of patients is its practical implementation. A key to the successful realisation of patients' rights is the emphasis placed on communication and understanding the reason why someone acts the way they do. It is also important to provide information to involved stakeholders about the existence of the law itself and its content. More important, however, is the need to communicate the underpinning values of patients' rights in terms of respect for the voice and choice of the individual citizen. Patient advocates and Patient Ombudsmen play an important role in communicating these critical messages. Sometimes lack of communication creates misunderstanding, which ends in a conflict between patients and health professionals. When this is the case, Patient Ombudsmen may act as mediators between the parties, or sometimes even as patients' advocates. The latter function of the Ombudsman is important in relation to the application of existing patients' rights. Often, Patient Ombudsmen play a role in applying the complaints procedure, either by taking responsibility for overseeing the complaints system, or being an integral part of such procedures.

The purpose of this book

The purpose of this book is to give a flavour of the experience of patient advocacy and Patient Ombudsman systems in seven European countries. The countries we have chosen are Austria, Finland, Greece, Hungary, Israel, Norway and the United Kingdom. All of them have used different avenues to approach the issue of promoting patients' rights and offering impartial investigations for citizens when alleged injustice has been committed in health services. A common denominator for the seven countries is the unbalanced relationship between patients and health professionals. By providing examples from countries with different values, levels of democracy, acceptance of patients' rights and legal traditions we want to encourage health professionals, health decision makers and other stakeholders to find new ways to reinforce existing patients' rights. It is our belief that the messages in this book can offer ideas for promoting and sustaining beneficial relationships between patients and health professionals and encourage a more active form of patient participation. We understand that it is difficult, if not impossible, to make a blueprint of a system in effect in one country and transfer it directly to another country. Instead we provide experiences of Patient Ombudsman systems in effect in a specific environment. It is our hope that some aspects of these experiences will prove to be useful in other countries.

The countries covered

The Patient Ombudsman systems presented cover a wide range of approaches. The Finnish system, with thousands of Ombudsmen working across the country, is significantly different from other systems in terms of the number of Ombudsmen employed and how they share their time working both as Ombudsmen and as health professionals. The Norwegian and Austrian Ombudsman systems have a different approach, with regional Patient Ombudsmen working full time. Moreover, in both Norway and Austria the Ombudsman function is perceived as being part of the regional complaints procedure and they claim to play an independent role in relation to healthcare. In the UK, Greece and Hungary, where national commissioners or Ombudsmen are in place, none of these institutions were originally set up to handle issues related to healthcare. However, as a result of later developments in that field, including an increasing need for an independent and impartial institution, healthcare services was added as an area in which these national institutions operate.

In the UK the function of Health Service Commissioner was later developed into being part of the overall complaints procedure covering public hospitals while the system in Greece and Hungary does not allow for competence in these institutions. Similarly, the work of the Hungarian Parliamentary Commissioner on Citizens' Rights was later backed up by the enactment of the General Health Act introducing patients' rights representatives active at the local and regional level. Israel is the only one of the seven countries included in this presentation where the National Patient Ombudsman has remained since the beginning. The power, role and function of the Israeli Ombudsman is similar to that of the British and Greece institutions, with the important difference that the Israeli Ombudsman is appointed directly by the Minister of Health and is backed up – formally – by regional health funds' Ombudsman officers and local patients' rights representatives.

Key introductory themes

At the start of this book, we set the scene with the notion of the Ombudsman coming into being: its origins in Sweden as a general system of administrative control and its expansion into the field of healthcare by Finland, the USA and the UK. Above all, it is in the context of what many regard as a basic set of human rights in healthcare, and a fundamental right to complain when those human rights are infringed, that the Ombudsman is set. Without a watchdog to ensure that procedures are followed to enable individuals to avail themselves of their rights as patients, the rights in themselves become useless. This is all the more important in the sphere of healthcare, where traditional subordination of the patient to the expertise of the clinician is reinforced, and complaints are therefore implicitly discouraged.

We went on to examine what the key features of that watchdog should be. First among these was impartiality: a requirement that should apply as a matter of ethics whether or not administrative and financial independence exists. Originally, the Ombudsman acted as an independent investigator, but in many countries, the role has changed, and it has become one of advocate for the patient's cause. Nevertheless, impartiality should remain at the heart of an Ombudsman's remit if s/he is to offer truly objective advice and support to patients.

Secondly, the staff exercising the functions of the Ombudsman need sufficient expertise to deal not only with the legal and administrative aspects of complaints, but also the highly technical and sensitive context of clinical care.

Thirdly, Ombudsmen should have powers which lend credibility and weight to their position and enable them to discharge their functions fully. Powers to sanction organisations which either fail to aid an Ombudsman's investigation or fail to act upon his/her recommendations are debatable. Too many, and the Ombudsman becomes another court, with all the cost and time that that entails. Too few, and the Ombudsman is a watchdog with no 'teeth'. However, procedural powers to carry out their duties to the full should abound. Principal among these is access to records – of any and all categories.

Fourthly, as a watchdog of due process, the Ombudsmen themselves should be rigorous in the systems they apply for investigating, reporting and recording cases. In respect of this final point, we proposed greater recognition for the role which the Ombudsman can play in contributing to quality improvement of health services more generally. Though caseloads may vary, depending on whether the Ombudsman is a local or a national entity, he or she can bring a unique perspective to the development of healthcare services which should not be undervalued.

How national systems compare

Systems appear to vary markedly from country to country. However, in each case, the role of the Ombudsman may be said to fall into one or more of the following categories, which reflect widely varying levels of responsibility and intervention:

- advice
- advocacy
- mediation
- arbitration.

Additionally, there appear to be clear areas within which patients in any given country will operate to try to satisfy their grievance. These can be said to fall along a continuum as follows:

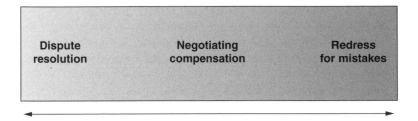

Figure 8.1 The role of the Ombudsman?

At one end of the spectrum, patients may have minor complaints or concerns which can be resolved informally within the health service provider organisation. Litigation, and indeed a protracted formal complaint, may rarely be involved. However, patients may need help and support to navigate the system and to obtain a result, formally or informally reached, which is mutually acceptable.

At the other end of the spectrum are the more serious grievances, for example of alleged clinical negligence and, in extreme cases, criminal activity. Patients may seek redress in the courts, or by demanding disciplinary proceedings against the clinician concerned. In either circumstance, when tackling the collective power of the professional fraternity the patient's interests need to be adequately represented and protected.

In between these two extremes, and overlapping with them to a certain extent, the question of compensation arises. In some countries, systems of no-fault compensation exist. These effectively mean that at the lower end of the scale, a patient's grievance may be resolved by a payment from a third party: the compensation fund. By contrast, patients seeking redress in the courts for clinical negligence will invariably be pleading for compensation as well as any other remedies which the court may grant.

The seven countries featured in this book demonstrate significant variations in the conceptualisation of the term 'Ombudsman'. These range from the local, and highly partisan, advocate, to national, statutorily independent investigator. In effect, the Ombudsman plays different roles in different countries which fall along the length of this continuum. Moreover, it is worth noting at this point that in a number of countries, a comprehensive approach has been adopted. That is to say that formally or informally the central role of an investigating, adjudicating Ombudsman has been supplemented with additional systems for advocacy and support for patients individually.

The legislation to promote patients' rights and the accompanying Ombudsman system have been well publicised in the Nordic region and beyond. In many ways they were ground-breaking, and are to be commended. However, the lack of real power, together with the compromising employment status of the Ombudsmen, give rise to justified criticism that the implementation of the patients' rights legislation in practice does not reflect the spirit and original intention of the law.

Nevertheless, this is recognised, and a clear case for reform and development has been made. In any reform, or introduction of such an institution, policymakers also need to be careful about whether they should adopt the title of 'Ombudsman' for the system they propose – and if so why. The range of systems outlined in this book shows that there can be confusion about the real nature of the Ombudsman. Where systems which rely exclusively on advocacy on the side of the patient are concerned, questions are raised as to whether they are truly Ombudsmen. Although purists would argue that a central parliamentary commissioner is the only real Ombudsman, we believe that in this modern day, there is no right answer. What is important is that the principles set out in this book, of impartiality, appropriate skills, sufficient powers and coherent systems, are fulfilled in any given example.

We shall now go on to consider the main features of each country, and where their principal advantages lie.

Austria

The Austrian Ombudsman system revolves around the provision of a statutory advocacy service for patients – the *Patientenanwalt*, derived from a more general-ised people's attorney, or *Volksanwalt*. These operate, uniquely, at a regional level, though supplemented in a few rare cases by voluntarily appointed hospital-based Ombudsmen. Patient advocates are statutorily independent, and by lifting them out of individual health institutions and providing funding from a separate public source, independence is clear and demonstrable.

The patient advocates benefit from a clear expectation of expertise in their chosen field. They also find themselves in the privileged position of being seen as largely unconfrontational in their advocacy: a statutory duty to seek extrajudicial settle-ment wherever possible, coupled with their association with a subsidised compen-sation scheme, promotes co-operative working with healthcare institutions.

Though evidence is anecdotal, the patient advocates appear by virtue of this position to be accorded a high degree of co-operation also in obtaining information in the course of case-handling. Public-sector healthcare providers, down to the level of individual clinicians, are statutorily obliged to provide information when requested. Private providers are not, but appear often to adhere to the same code voluntarily. Nevertheless, it is not clear what the true extent of this co-operation is, or what sanctions could be invoked for non-co-operation by a public sector provider.

Devolution of responsibility to a regional level, together with the limited term of office for any individual advocate, have also resulted in a degree of fragmentation in terms of record-keeping, consistency, and ways of working. A loose represen-tative confederation of the *Patientenanwalt* has been formed, with a goal of shared learning and promotion of the patients' rights agenda as a whole. However, the circumstances of devolution militate against the Ombudsman system as a cohesive national force for change and improvement. This is an area all the more ripe for action given the existing responsibility felt by the *Patientenanwalt* for acting as a safeguard for quality.

Finland

The Ombudsman in Finland represents perhaps the most devolved and restricted system in this book. It consists of a network of some 2000 individuals, acting as advisers to patients within local healthcare institutions at municipality level. The system springs from a national drive to promote and support patients' rights as a whole. This is evident most plainly in the explicit legislation passed to underpin patients' rights, and the associated obligation on local healthcare providers to have a Patient Ombudsman working within their institution.

Curiously, however, the individuals acting as Ombudsmen are largely part-time appointees. For the rest of their time they are for the most part employees of those institutions, working as social workers or nurses. Independence and the question of conflict of interest are therefore uppermost in any assessment of this system. These individuals are under a duty to act impartially, and do not at any time act as advocates for patients, rather investigating complaints as intermediaries between provider and patient. However, their ability to act as a force for improvement is heavily curtailed by the absence of powers or skills. These Ombudsmen appear largely to be providers of information. There is no minimum skills set or basic training for Ombudsmen appointees, and the role seems to be very much secondary to their 'day job'.

Powers to investigate are unclear but, critically, there is no power to make recommendations for change as a result. The localised nature of the work and variations in practice also mean that there is little comparative data available nationally to assess or compare the activities of the 2000 Ombudsmen in Finland.

Greece

Though springing from a phrase literally translated as a citizen's advocate, the Greek system reflects the more traditional concept of the Ombudsman as a centrally based mediator and investigator. The importance of the Ombudsman in Greece as a public sector-wide service is reinforced by the sheer size and scale of public administration. Democratic freedom was hard fought, but the resulting governmental machine is heavily politicised. In this context the Ombudsman has been a relatively recent response to the inadequacy of traditional means of redress for individual citizens.

The resulting office of Ombudsman is therefore explicitly and statutorily independent, and appears well structured and provided for, with a specific arm dealing with healthcare and social welfare sector grievances. This arm benefits from a team of investigators with a wide range of appropriate clinical and legal expertise, although medical advice needs largely to be commissioned at this stage in the form of expert opinion. *Prima facie* the Ombudsman also has wide-ranging powers of investigation, with statutory provision for access to records and summoning witnesses.

What is less clear is the ability of the Ombudsman to enforce these powers. This is perhaps highlighted by the fact that data about the Ombudsman's activities are as yet scarce. The office of Ombudsman has only been in place for four or five years. Couple this with a still heavily paternalistic model of healthcare where individuals are reluctant to question or complain. Healthcare therefore represents only a small portion of the Ombudsman's workload as a whole, and there is still much to be done to raise public awareness of the system and its potential.

The small caseload and the newness of the patients' rights agenda also militate against the Ombudsman acting as a powerful force for quality improvement of the healthcare system generally at this stage. It is early days, however, and the Ombudsman has already commissioned an evaluation of systems and operations to date. Given this zeal for self-improvement, and the strong statutory footing which the Ombudsman has been given, the system has a great deal of potential for the future.

Hungary

The Hungarian model of Ombudsman function, like that of the UK, stems first and foremost from the notion of a central, statutory, parliamentary watchdog. This is a parliamentary commissioner, displaying very much the traditional range of investigative powers, with powers to sanction and penalise absent. Uniquely, the Hungarian Parliamentary Commissioner's sphere of competence appears to be categorised according to types of human rights, with a series of commissioners with expertise in areas such as minority rights and data protection. There is no specific competence in the field of healthcare, but where human rights and the rights of patients overlap, then the Ombudsman can and does investigate.

The interesting development which has come to supplement this system has been the emphasis on introducing new legislation to underpin the rights of patients, and the subsequent introduction of local patients' rights representatives. These are statutory appointees, independently employed, with expertise in patients' rights and powers to investigate, interview and to access records and premises. They are also empowered to make recommendations for change as a result of complaints, and to keep healthcare staff informed of the nature and scope of patients' rights.

As in some other countries, therefore, there has been a gradual proliferation to all levels of the system. This means providing local, impartial support advocacy and advice, up to national, statutorily independent investigation of grievances. Both the national Ombudsman and the local patient representatives appear to be well used mechanisms by the Hungarian public. The role of the patients' rights representatives has yet to be evaluated, and there is an absence of aggregated data about their work and functions. However, if anything it is these local advocates who have the power and the position to influence improvements in the way services are configured and delivered, at least at a local level.

Israel

The Israeli approach to legislating for an Ombudsman is one of the most legislatively comprehensive in the world. In contrast to the UK, where there is a traditional reliance on informal or conventional mechanisms to supplement basic statutory obligations, Israel has chosen to legislate for an Ombudsman at all levels. A central Health Insurance Ombudsman is complemented by a statutory obligation on each of the private health fund providers to appoint an internal Ombudsman responsible for safeguarding patients' rights and investigating complaints; and by a duty on each health institution locally to designate a local Ombudsman acting as patients' rights representative.

The system is comprehensive in its coverage (applying in a series of tiers from national to highly localised), in its accessibility (allowing direct access for complainants to any level of the system), in its powers of investigation and in its support for individuals (providing both advocacy and investigative dispute resolution). This must be measured against the absence of any defined skills sets guaranteeing the quality of any given Ombudsman's work.

In addition, akin to the problems of co-ordination created by regional devolution in Austria, the fragmentation of the system to various levels has resulted in a loss of co-ordination and consistency. More critically, the nature of the role and employment terms of the health fund and local Ombudsmen gives rise to concerns about conflicts of interest. Impartiality may be assured in the letter of the law, and perhaps by the ethics of the individuals concerned, but true independence cannot be demonstrated.

Norway

For much the same reasons as in Greece the office of Ombudsman in Norway was created originally as a national institution in the face of a vast public administration. The concept has since been expanded into the field of healthcare with a team of county level Patient Ombudsmen. These offices sprang up originally from grass roots, however, and there were – and still are – variations in roles and responsibilities despite more recent legislative co-ordination.

Historically, the skills sets of these local officers also vary, as do their attitudes to the role. They operate, and are clearly independent, but the role represents a curious amalgamation of a number of tasks which in other countries are performed by different bodies. In Norway the Patient Ombudsman is seen as an informal mediator, who can have recourse to more formal investigation and adjudication, and also an officer who may support and advise a patient in pursuing an alternative course of complaint.

This amalgam of roles appears to work well, however, with neutrality and independence still remaining at the forefront. While no national level evaluation has been undertaken yet, local evaluations demonstrate a high degree of support for, and satisfaction with, the Patient Ombudsman, among both patients and healthcare professionals. More importantly, healthcare staff themselves cite the Ombudsman as a driver in improving internal controls for quality and safety. Indeed, it appears that hospital management do invite the Patient Ombudsman to contribute to quality improvement exercises. This is an emerging aspect of their role, however. There is still a need to achieve a minimum level of expertise – particularly in legal training – and uniformity of practice across the country.

The Patient Ombudsmen have various statutory powers to interview and gain access to records, obtaining information even from healthcare providers outside the Ombudsman's decision-making jurisdiction. They cannot impose real sanctions directly for failure to comply by a healthcare provider, but remain very powerful implicitly: there is always the option of forwarding a case to the County Medical Officer, who has the legal power of sanction, or the right to make their opinion public ('naming and shaming' the obstructive body or individual). As a result, recommendations are seldom not followed in practice, and healthcare providers do as a rule see the Ombudsman's existence as a positive.

The national parliamentary commissioner seems to have only very marginal dealings with healthcare, only a minimal number of complaints being received at this level. By contrast, the Patient Ombudsman scheme is extremely well used. The Patient Ombudsman has an express objective of driving local quality improvement (though this is secondary to the primary function of protecting and promoting patients' rights). There is an explicit statutory duty too for them to publicise their findings, which often receive attention from the press, and they will become more powerful from this year when national aggregated data will become available from a shared database.

They are not yet seen as on quite the same social footing as the general parliamentary commissioner, but have benefited by association, and need now to consolidate their position by continuing to raise awareness of their role and impact.

United Kingdom

The UK has adopted the traditional notion of the Ombudsman as a statutorily independent, nationally based investigator. Initial general parliamentary functions gave rise to a subsequent specific expansion into healthcare.

Interestingly, akin to developments in Israel and Hungary, the statutory system is backed up by a range of formal and informal mechanisms which provide the direct local advocacy support which patients need. These include:

- a patient advice and liaison service, employed within each healthcare institution, providing guidance about grievance procedures, and acting on the spot to resolve potential complaints informally
- a statutorily independent complaints advocacy service, for patients wishing to register a formal complaint.

Within this sphere, the Ombudsman occupies a position well backed up by powers to summon witnesses and to access records, breaches of which can be treated as akin to contempt of court. The sanctions remain procedural, however, and do not extend as far as a substantive power to enforce recommendations. The system is also well supported by the existence of a directorate of expert clinical advisers, ensuring that the currency and skill of the Ombudsman's office is maintained.

However, the relatively small caseload calls into question the Ombudsman's ability, alone, to review and shape quality improvement generally. However, the overarching nature of the role, the methods of investigation at the Ombudsman's disposal, and the unique perspective which that position offers make the findings of the Ombudsman – specific and generic – highly persuasive in assessing the future development of services.

Conclusions and final remarks

The experiences from Patient Ombudsmen systems presented above point out some key areas to be borne in mind when introducing future systems to deal with patients who are dissatisfied with the care and treatment they have received. As one would expect, principles such as impartiality, appropriate skill and powers and good support systems must be observed when developing new systems. As we have seen in some reports, the degree of bureaucracy in a country and the existence of other institutions with similar functions might create difficulties as to the competence and jurisdiction of a Patient Ombudsman function and that of existing institutions.

National and local Ombudsman functions

One important dilemma is whether a Patient Ombudsman system should be organised nationally or regionally/locally. On closer inspection of the Israeli and Hungarian systems it is quite clear that the existence and work of the local patient representatives simplify the work of the national Ombudsman. Having knowledge of local working procedures, routines and developments makes it easier to suggest improvements and monitor changes when a local unit has been criticised. Similarly, a national Ombudsman plays an important role in co-ordinating the work going on across the country and can feed back experiences and examples of good practice where it is needed, particularly from the perspective of national policy reform. The national Ombudsman and the regional Ombudsmen in Israel are not legally required to collaborate. The same situation is in place in Hungary. However, in Israel Ombudsmen from both levels meet informally to share experiences and methods and to solve problems.

In Finland and Norway, where systems with local and regional Ombudsmen are in effect, it is clear that there is a need for a central body with responsibility to collect and disseminate information. Facing similar problems and being geographically spread out over a large area makes it necessary to be more effective in problem solving and reviewing cases. Standardising the handling of complaints and systematising the process for recording outcomes and reporting will probably make the Ombudsmen more effective. Moreover, a central Ombudsman might be in a better position to make judgements as to what resources are needed in different areas.

Local knowledge and quality improvement

Several authors in this book point out the need for the Ombudsman to share knowledge and experience with health services. It is difficult to argue against such an approach when one of the aims of the Ombudsman system is to improve overall healthcare quality. As stated in, for example, § 8-2 of the Norwegian Act on the rights of patients, 'The patient ombud shall work to safeguard patients' rights, interests and legal rights in their relations with the health service and to improve the quality of the health service.' When analysing the question more thoroughly, however, some problems arise. Firstly, local knowledge is important when sharing experience and providing support in the local quality improvement process. Knowledge about organisational development, who is really in charge, who has the 'real' say in quality improvement issues, for example, are critical. Secondly, to enable the Ombudsman to be effective, it is important that the law explicitly describes how the experience and knowledge of the Ombudsman shall be communicated, for example by having a seat in the local quality committee etc. If the provision is of a more general nature, it is fairly easy to ignore such legislation by referring to more stifled forms of communication, such as the sharing of written documents. Thirdly, as stated in the chapter describing the British system, it is important to have enough complaints to be able to express a valid opinion. This makes it difficult for national Ombudsmen with a low number of cases and limited local knowledge about the health services to be effective in terms of quality improvement on a local and/or regional level.

The power of the Patient Ombudsman

In some of the chapters of this book the Patient Ombudsman is described as an additional institution through which patients can launch a complaint. This is, of course, positive from the point of view of the patient, who is given an additional route to complain to those already available. However, when analysing existing systems to monitor the quality and standard of health professionals and health-care units a recurring problem is the tension between the health inspectorate (or similar) on the one side, and the health professionals on the other. The fear of being reported or accused of malpractice is frequently mentioned as an obstacle for quality improvement. As an example, in Sweden (a system not represented in this book) health professionals have to report to the National Board of Health and Welfare when there is a risk that a patient will be injured, or when patients in fact have been injured because of mistakes in health services. This information is gathered in a national database and is analysed and fed back to the health professionals across the country. However, the National Board of Health and Welfare is obliged to report any health professional to the disciplinary board if it suspects that he/she is responsible for causing a patient injury. The risk of being reported makes it difficult to collect data and the number of unreported cases is estimated at as high as 95%.

One advantage of the Patient Ombudsman system is that this institution is not empowered to sanction health professionals or impose fines. However, the professional judgement of the Ombudsman to report the case to the appropriate authorities or to put pressure on an organisation or unit to improve their procedures might be even more effective. This way the Patient Ombudsman will be perceived by health professionals as someone whose aim is to improve overall quality. More-over, it might simplify the collection of preventive data if health professionals do not feel they stand the risk of being reported if they voluntarily share experiences of mistakes made or similar.

It is, however, also possible to argue that an Ombudsman institution lacking the right to impose sanctions or fines will be ineffective. Following this line of argument makes the existence of 'teeth' necessary if one wants to create real change. This problem is probably related to the context in which the Ombudsman is expected to work. While in some environments the use of threats to sanction and impose fines is necessary, other systems are more sensitive in responding to public criticism or public investigations.

Gate keeping by local complaint resolution?
In 1996 the British government decided to accept the Wilson Committee's recommendation for a two-stage complaints procedure. In practice, this means that patients are expected to use all locally available means to resolve their grievance by using local or regional complaints procedures before they can turn to the Health Service Commissioner with their complaint. As described by Giddings, complainants do still have direct access to the HSC. This is however limited by the decision of the commissioner and whether he/she is of the opinion that local and regional complaints procedures have been 'invoked and exhausted'. From the perspective of any government it is more time effective and cost effective to 'push' complainants towards local complaint resolution. This way resources will not be tied up in 'unnecessary' cases that could have been resolved locally. Having several complaints procedures available increases the risk that patients launch complaints to all of them at the same time without any thought as to what remedies can be available from each.

Looking at the problem from the other side, any limitation of a patient's right to launch a complaint to the Ombudsmen is a serious curtailment. In the British example, the rights of patients to direct access to the Health Service Commissioner is decided by the commissioner. Of course it could be argued that the commissioner will oversee the whole complaints procedure and whether it is used in an effective way. But what if resources are scarce and the commissioner refuses to review complaints owing to a lack of resources (rather than because all possibilities to complain have not been 'invoked and exhausted')? When such a serious limitation as preventing direct access to the commissioner is in effect, it is important that the activities and decisions of the commissioner about whether or not to pursue a case are evaluated by external resources.

The ideal Patient Ombudsman scheme

If there is such a thing as an ideal Patient Ombudsman scheme we would like to believe that its work develops hand in hand with the expectations of citizens and the respect of health professionals. The work of the Patient Ombudsman is a delicate balance for any institution in any country. Pressure groups will of course influence the activities of an Ombudsman in a way that is beneficial to them. Therefore, to be credible, it is important for the Ombudsman to act in way that will not expose the office to criticism of a kind that might be perceived as biased towards a particular group. Independence and impartiality are key words, although the extent of the definitions applied to each could be debated for some time. However, the best way to prove that the decisions taken by the Ombudsman are justified is by its acceptance from different stakeholders and the continued confidence in the Ombudsman function. Following the experiences from the seven countries presented in this book we believe that future Ombudsman schemes should include the following features:

- standardised systems with regard to the handling, systematising and reporting of the complaints (local Ombudsmen)
- comprise full-time employed officers with no conflicting interests
- reports or investigations made by the Ombudsman should be made public
- the Ombudsman institution should be regulated by law, including a prerequisite basic skills set for the staff and the role of the Ombudsman in local quality improvement
- the jurisdiction of the Ombudsman should include the care and treatment of inpatients as well as outpatients
- regular evaluation of the activities of the Ombudsman should be carried out independently
- there should be no limitation of the Ombudsman's power to access documents or evidence regarded as relevant by the Ombudsman
- the Ombudsman should monitor any complaints procedures in existence.

Finally we would like to encourage decision-makers in countries with a strong commitment to the protection of patients' rights to develop their own Patient Ombudsman schemes. There are a myriad of considerations to make on the way to developing a system to specific domestic circumstances, and it is useful to try a system on a smaller scale, drawing on the experience of other countries such as those covered in this book, before committing wholly to a particular model.

Index